D0002678

Occupational Adaptation
in Practice

Concepts and Cases

Janette Schkade
Melissa McClung

SLACK Incorporated

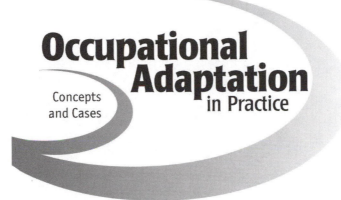

Occupational
Adaptation
in Practice

Concepts and Cases

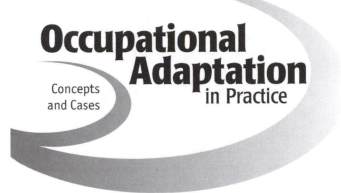

Occupational Adaptation

Adaptation

Concepts and Cases

in Practice

Janette Schkade, PhD, OTR, FAOTA
School of Occupational Therapy
Texas Woman's University
Denton, Texas

Melissa McClung, MOT, OTR
School of Occupational Therapy
Texas Woman's University
Denton, Texas

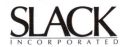

an innovative information, education, and management company
6900 Grove Road • Thorofare, NJ 08086

BELMONT UNIVERSITY LIBRARY

Copyright © 2001 by SLACK Incorporated

All rights reserved. No part of this book may be reproduced, stored in a retrieval system or transmitted in any form or by any means, electronic, mechanical, photocopying, recording or otherwise, without written permission from the publisher, except for brief quotations embodied in critical articles and reviews.

The procedures and practices described in this book should be implemented in a manner consistent with the professional standards set for the circumstances that apply in each specific situation. Every effort has been made to confirm the accuracy of the information presented and to correctly relate generally accepted practices. The author, editor, and publisher cannot accept responsibility for errors or exclusions or for the outcome of the application of the material presented herein. There is no expressed or implied warranty of this book or information imparted by it. Any review or mention of specific companies or products is not intended as an endorsement by the author or the publisher.

The work SLACK publishes is peer reviewed. Prior to publication, recognized leaders in the field, educators, and clinicians provide important feedback on the concepts and content that we publish. We welcome feedback on this work.

Schkade, Janette K.
    Occupational adaptation in practice : concepts and cases / Janette K. Schkade, Melissa McClung.
        p. ; cm.
    Includes bibliographical references and index.
    ISBN 1-55642-553-8 (alk. paper)
        1. Occupational therapy--Handbooks, manuals, etc. 2. Occupational therapy--Case studies. I. McClung, Melissa, II. Title.
RM735.3 .S35 2001
615.8'515--dc21   2001042910

Printed in the United States of America
Published by: SLACK Incorporated
                      6900 Grove Road
                      Thorofare, NJ 08086 USA
                      Telephone: 856-848-1000
                      Fax: 856-853-5991
                      www.slackbooks.com

Contact SLACK Incorporated for more information about other books in this field or about the availability of our books from distributors outside the United States.

Authorization to photocopy items for internal or personal use, or the internal or personal use of specific clients, is granted by SLACK Incorporated, provided that the appropriate fee is paid directly to Copyright Clearance Center, 222 Rosewood Drive, Danvers, MA 01923 USA, 978-750-8400. Prior to photocopying items for educational classroom use, please contact the CCC at the address above. Please reference Account Number 9106324 for SLACK Incorporated's Professional Book Division.

For further information on CCC, check CCC Online at the following address: http://www.copyright.com.

Last digit is print number: 10 9 8 7 6 5 4 3 2 1

BELMONT UNIVERSITY LIBRARY

RM
735.3
.S35
2001

202134

DEDICATION

To those practitioners and students who have brought occupational adaptation to life through their skillful, thoughtful, and client-centered interventions, we dedicate this book.

CONTENTS

Dedication v
About the Authors ix
Preface xi
Before You Begin xv

Chapter One.   **What is Occupational Adaptation?** **1**
Concept: overview of occupational adaptation theory

Case: Jill *3*

Chapter Two.   **How Do the Person and Environment Relate?** **13**
Concepts: desire for mastery, demand for mastery,
and press for mastery

Case: The Afghan Maker *17*
Try it On *19*

Chapter Three.   **How Do Occupational Role Expectations Fit in?** ..**21**
Concepts: occupational challenge, internal and
external expectations, person and occupational
environment

Case: The Water Skier *27*
Try it On *28*

Chapter Four.   **How Does the Person Begin to Produce the
Response?** **31**
Concept: the adaptive response generation sub-
process (adaptive response mechanism)

Case: The Preacher *38*
Case: The Researcher *40*
Case: The Chess Player *43*
Try it On *47*

Chapter Five.   **What's the Plan to Carry Out the Response?** **51**
Concept: the adaptive response generation sub-
process (adaptation gestalt)

Case: The Husband Caregiver *54*
Try it On *57*

Chapter Six.   **What's Right or Wrong With This Picture?** **61**
Concept: the adaptive response evaluation sub-
process (relative mastery)

Case: The Florist *64*
Try it On *66*

Chapter Seven.   **How Has the Person Changed or Adapted?** **69**
Concept: the adaptive response integration
subprocess

Case: The Elder Homemaker *72*
Try it On *74*

Chapter Eight.   **How Does the Environment Respond?** **77**
Concepts: assessment by the occupational
environment and incorporation by the occupational
environment

Try it On *82*

Chapter Nine.   **What Does the Therapist Do?** **85**
Case: The Pianist *88*
Case: The Woodworker *90*

Chapter Ten.   **How Do You Describe Occupational Adaptation
to Others?** **93**

Index *101*

About the Authors

Janette Schkade, after graduating with a PhD in psychology, practiced as a psychologist in a state school for the mentally challenged, working with clients who had multiple physical as well as mental disabilities. It was in this environment that she learned about occupational therapy and what it could do for this population. She then obtained her education in occupational therapy from Texas Woman's University. She is a co-author of the Occupational Adaptation Theoretical Framework. She has presented at national and regional conferences on this framework, both as theory and as a vehicle to guide practice. She is the author or co-author of numerous publications regarding occupational adaptation, both in scholarly journals and book chapters.

Melissa McClung has been practicing with the occupational adaptation theoretical perspective for 10 years. She has had the opportunity to use the theory in practice with patients, in redesigning existing occupational therapy programs, and in student programs in clinic settings—most currently in classroom curriculum design/implementation as a faculty member at Texas Woman's University, Denton. She has presented her approach to occupational adaptation at national and regional conferences. Prior to becoming an occupational therapist, she practiced as a music therapist for 8 years.

PREFACE

Occupational therapy practitioners often complain that theory is not useful. A common perception is that theory is just for the classroom and not for the clinic. An associated belief is that theory limits what one can do in practice and therefore should be avoided in therapeutic situations in favor of doing "what works."

We disagree with those ideas. We instead believe that theory is extremely useful in guiding a practice that is versatile, effective, and efficient. However, the usefulness of theory depends on the therapist having a working understanding of the principles. A thorough understanding enables the therapist to be creative and responsive to the dynamic needs of the client. The purpose of this book is to make occupational adaptation understandable and useful.

Occupational adaptation, a theoretical frame of reference, was developed as part of a planning process for the PhD in Occupational Therapy program at Texas Woman's University. The conceptual framework was designed for two equally important purposes. First, it was to provide a research focus for the program; second, it was to be a guide for therapeutic intervention. It first appeared in print in a two-part article (Schkade & Schultz, 1992; Schultz & Schkade, 1992). The format of the articles was specifically designed with the practitioner in mind. The intention was for therapists to find it useful in guiding their thinking and in articulating to others what they were doing in the practice of occupational therapy.

Numerous workshops and presentations at regional and national conferences have attempted to further explain the framework (both as a description of "normal" occupational function and as a way of thinking about dysfunctional occupational function). However, many therapists attending those events have expressed a need for additional aids in understanding and therapeutically applying the frame of reference. This book grew out of a desire to make the occupational adaptation frame of reference more understandable and easier to use clinically. We hope we have succeeded in this purpose.

We are grateful to the therapists who have shared their therapeutic work in the form of cases that appear in this book. These cases are powerful examples of the advantages to be gained by both client and therapist when a holistic approach centered on the client's preferred occupations guides intervention. There are other theory-based approaches to intervention, which are available to the practitioner, that are client-centered and occupation-focused. Law (1998), in her book on client-focused intervention, names several. Occupational adaptation is not the only approach. The therapist who finds another perspective effective in producing desired results with clients is encouraged to continue use of that satisfying method. For the therapist who is seeking to expand a therapeutic repertoire or is seeking a way of making intervention more holistic and client-centered, we hope that this guide, with its cases and the suggested readings, will provide assistance in that endeavor.

The guide is organized following occupational adaptation depicted in the basic process figure in Chapter One (Figure 1-1).* Each chapter describes one of the theoretical ideas in language that we hope will be understandable. We have described these ideas both in terms of "normative" occupational functioning as well as in given cases in which therapists have engaged patients who were experiencing occupational dysfunction.

In addition to the cases, each chapter has a feature designed to help bring the ideas to life. This feature is called "Try it On." It suggests ways in which you can apply the ideas to your own life. We believe that occupational adaptation is a capability present in all human beings. Our experience has been that the therapists who use this frame of reference in practice most effectively have applied it to their own lives and found that it made sense. We invite you to do the same through the "Try it On" feature in this book.

Chapter One presents an overview of the theory. Chapters Two through Eight are an explanation of the theory with cases and the "Try it On" feature. Chapter Nine discusses what the therapist does to use occupational adaptation in practice. Chapter Ten is called "How Do You Describe Occupational Adaptation to Others?" This chapter helps those who are trying to explain the framework to others. Maybe you have to provide an inservice to fellow therapists about occupational adaptation. Maybe you are a supervisor of fieldwork students or a faculty member instructing students in the clinic or classroom. This chapter contains methods we have found to be useful in such teaching situations. We hope you will find these examples useful as well.

Most of all, we hope that this book will reinforce what you do as occupational therapists. We hope it will increase your commitment to, your enjoyment of, and your excitement about the practice of client-centered occupational therapy.

References

Law, M. (1998). *Client-centered occupational therapy.* Thorofare, NJ: SLACK Incorporated.

Schkade, J. K. & Schultz, S. (1992). Occupational adaptation: Toward a holistic approach to contemporary practice, Part 1. *Am J Occup Ther, 46,* 829-837.

Schultz, S. & Schkade, J. K. (1992). Occupational adaptation: Toward a holistic approach to contemporary practice, Part 2. *Am J Occup Ther, 46,* 917-926.

*Figure 1-1, as well as adaptations of it throughout the book, is reprinted with permission from Schkade, J. & Schultz, S. (1992). Occupational adaptation: Toward a holistic approach for contemporary practice. Part 1. *Am J Occup Ther, 46,* 832. © The American Occupational Therapy Association, Inc.

Before You Begin

A Few Words About Theory in General
- Theory is made up of concepts.
  That's why it can be hard to understand at first.
- Theory describes relationships between the concepts.
  These relationships are the "glue" that links the pieces together.
- Each theory has a unique terminology.
  The key to understanding any theory is to become comfortable with the terminology.

A Few Words About the Theory of Occupational Adaptation
- Occupational adaptation describes a "normal" process.
  You will see the flow of this "normal" process in a basic diagram.
- This process can become disrupted during periods of transition or stress.
  Disruption can lead to dysfunction.
- Restoration of this process is the goal of intervention.
  Skill acquisition is not the focus. The client's capacity to engage in preferred life roles is the goal.

A Few Words About How This Book is Designed to Promote Understanding of the Theory of Occupational Adaptation
- Each chapter focuses on a separate occupational adaptation concept.
  Concepts are described to illustrate both function and dysfunction.
- Therapist-reported cases enhance understanding.
  These cases are strategically placed in the book as examples of occupational adaptation concepts in practice.
- A "Try it On" feature in most chapters enhances understanding through personal application.
  This feature has been designed to have the reader apply occupational adaptation to a personal situation. The reader will use the same personal situation throughout the book.

CHAPTER ONE

What is Occupational Adaptation

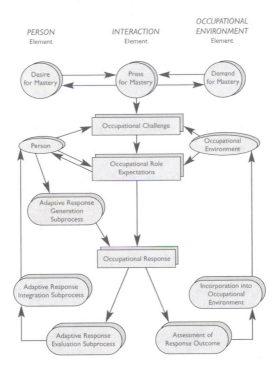

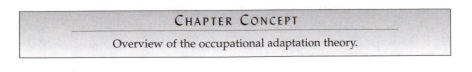

CHAPTER CONCEPT

Overview of the occupational adaptation theory.

What is occupational adaptation? It is basically two things:
1. It is a concept that describes a human phenomenon.
2. It is a framework that therapists can use to guide their intervention planning and implementation.

Occupational adaptation as it was first articulated in Schkade and Schultz (1992) and Schultz and Schkade (1992) is one description of a process that is thought to be present in all human beings. That process exists in humans to allow us to respond masterfully and adaptively to the various occupational challenges that we encounter over a lifetime. We believe that this process provides the tools that humans need to develop and sustain competence in carrying out the tasks associated with the various life roles we take on—in other words, competence in occupational functioning.

Life roles provide the context for expressing our competence in occupational functioning. The occupational adaptation process provides the systems for carrying out those roles adaptively and masterfully. The tasks contained in life roles change from time to time, requiring us to adapt in order to be successful. We also believe that demand on the occupational adaptation process is greatest when the individual must transition to changing life roles. The greater the transition, the more at risk this process is for disruption. For example, a person with a spinal cord injury faces a major life transition in areas of occupational functioning such as work, leisure, and self-care. If that person's occupational adaptation process is functioning marginally, it is most likely to become dysfunctional under such extreme challenge. If, as we suggest, this process is the means by which we develop and sustain competence in occupational functioning, then it seems logical that a healthy process is most likely to result in meeting the challenges. This process facilitates development of life skills that must be adapted to the new or reduced capabilities. Therefore, the repair or restoration of the process is critical. The therapist who practices using this framework thus intervenes from the assumption that the therapeutic task is to facilitate a healthy occupational adaptation process in the client. This point of view empowers the client to be his or her own agent of competence development. The therapist simply, but very importantly, sets the stage for this process to unfold and function at its best.

It is important to recognize that the occupational adaptation process is a "normative" process. That means that it is not just something that operates in people who have experienced disease, trauma, or stress. It operates in you and me. At one time or another, each of us has been occupationally dysfunctional. Some of us have been so more frequently or for longer periods of time than others have been, but we have all experienced this dysfunction. This is why we recommend that a therapist wishing to use this perspective in intervention should first "try it on" with regard to his or her own life role adaptation challenges. If it seems to "fit," then the therapist will have an understanding of the practical application of the theory and adaptation process and, thus, be much better equipped to use it as a guide to intervention. If it does not seem to have some kind of practical validity, using it in practice with a sufficient understanding to intervene effectively may be more difficult. The story of Jill offers one example of how the need for individuals to adapt in ordinary life circumstances can appear.

JILL

We will illustrate this normative process through the transition of Jill to the role of first-time mother. Jill is a physically active person with a high activity level. She thinks things through and enjoys making lists for her day's tasks. Jill is elated with motherhood, enjoys being a homemaker, and feels content after a full day of successfully completed activities. Jill enters motherhood desiring a well cared for and loved baby while keeping an organized home and meeting her husband's needs. She lives in a two-bedroom apartment with her husband of 5 years, Jack. By mutual consent, Jack is the primary "bread winner" of the family. On this particular day, based on her activity list, Jill's plans include taking care of and spending quality time with her baby, cleaning her house, cooking a nutritious meal for her and Jack, and picking up Jack's suit at the dry cleaners for his business meeting tomorrow. Jill attacks the day ahead with exuberant amounts of energy; however, her "system" for cleaning house is interrupted by a gassy and fussy baby. Thus, by evening, Jack arrives home to a partially cleaned home, no prepared dinner, and no dry-cleaned suit. Jill is frustrated by the day's events, as is Jack. Jill makes a mental note to try the same method tomorrow and try harder.

Jill's decision to try the same plan again that did not work the first time reflects how in normal life transitions, we may fail to adapt even though there is a need for adaptation. Jill may wind up repeating this dysfunctional pattern more than once before she perceives any need for adaptation. Jill's occupational adaptation process will have to be more functional if she is to experience success in her new role.

The day in Jill's life that was just described can be thought of in terms of the occupational adaptation process. Figure 1-1 is a visual representation of this process.

Figure 1-1 represents a "cross-section" taken from the process that is stopped in time in order for us to look at the concepts and their relationships more closely. This is an artificial "freeze-frame" approach, much as one sees in a CT scan cross-section of the brain or spine. You can see the structures and note some relationships with regard to proximity and appearance. However, the image on the scan does not convey the dynamic nature of the ways in which these structures interact in routine functioning. The same thing is true of the occupational adaptation process figure. In real time, the process may be proceeding very rapidly and the individual will likely be dealing with multiple challenges at the same time or sometimes in quick succession. Our discussion in the subsequent chapters will also "stop" the process so that you can examine it more closely and thereby gain a deeper understanding of the concepts, their relationships, and the flow of the process.

The purpose of this book is to facilitate understanding of the occupational adaptation process and to make it therapeutically useful. Chapters are organized around the components of the process as seen in Figure 1-1. We will refer to this figure often during our discussion. **In each chapter where a concept is introduced, it will appear in italics as the concept is repeated in the discussion.** This will help you to develop an easy familiarity with the language of occupational adaptation. Explanations of each component will be followed by case examples contributed by therapists who have used this framework in practice.

There are important principles of intervention to keep in mind as you read the chapters. These principles are seen in Table 1-1. If you do not understand the terms at first glance, don't worry. The remaining chapters and case descriptions will bring them to life through skillful application by therapists with actual clients.

A therapist intervening with occupational adaptation must remember three "essentials" as the therapeutic process unfolds:

1. Your client will more likely achieve his or her goals if the internal adaptation process is working well. As with any intervention plan, revisions may be necessary if the adaptation process is not responding well to the plan and client goals are not being met.

2. There are three constant factors present in this process:
    - The person desires to function masterfully and adaptively
    - The occupational environment demands mastery of the person
    - The interaction of the desire for mastery and the demand for mastery produces the press for mastery

    If your client does not demonstrate this desire, you cannot assume

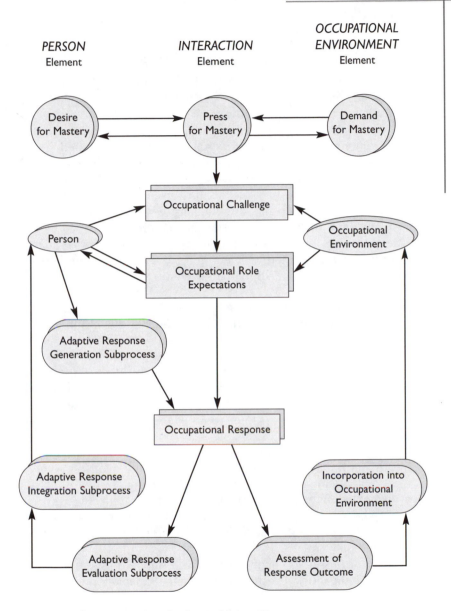

Figure 1-1. The occupational adaptation process.

Table 1-1

GUIDING PRINCIPLES FOR INTERVENTION

1. Occupational adaptation is not a collection of techniques but a way of directing the therapist's thinking about intervention in the individual's internal adaptation process.
2. Intervention is guided not by concerns about skill development but by the requirements of an occupational role that is identified by the client as meaningful. This role takes place within an environmental context about which the client or family must educate the therapist. Evaluation of strengths and deficits in sensorimotor, cognitive, and psychosocial systems is measured against what promotes or inhibits the client's ability to carry out the meaningful role.
3. A personally meaningful intervention focused on the internal adaptation process will be more efficient and the outcomes more likely to generalize to other contexts than intervention focused on general skill development.
4. Intervention is a combination of methods:
   • Occupational readiness is designed to address deficits in the sensorimotor, cognitive, and/or psychosocial systems. These interventions prepare or ready these systems to engage in occupation.
   • Occupational activities simulate or replicate tasks of the meaningful occupational role that will guide intervention and that will direct the focus on the client's internal adaptation process. These activities must meet the three required properties for occupations: active participation by the client, meaning to the client, and process ending in a tangible or intangible product.
5. The client evaluates his or her progress in terms of relative mastery:
   • Use of time, energy, and resources (efficiency)
   • Extent to which the desired goal was achieved (effectiveness)
   • Degree to which the personal actions producing the outcome were personally and socially well-regarded (satisfaction to self and society)
6. The therapist assesses client progress with standard assessment tools and with indications that the client's internal adaptation process has been affected:
   • Spontaneous generalization to other activities
   • Initiation of new approaches in novel situations
   • Increase in relative mastery

Reprinted with permission from Schultz, S. & Schkade, J. (1997). Adaptation. In C. Christiansen & C. Baum (Eds.), *Occupational Therapy, Enabling Function and Well-Being. (2nd Ed.)*, p. 476. Thorofare, NJ: SLACK Incorporated.

Table 1-2

OCCUPATIONAL ADAPTATION GUIDE TO PRACTICE

Occupational Adaptation Data Gathering/Assessment

What are the patient's *occupational environments* and *roles*?

Which role is of primary concern to patient and family?

What occupational performance is expected in the primary *occupational environment* and *role*?

What are the *physical, social,* and *cultural* features of the primary *occupational environment* and *role*?

What is the patient's *sensorimotor, cognitive,* and *psychosocial* status?

What is the patient's level of *relative mastery* in the primary *occupational environment* and *role*?

What is facilitating or limiting *relative mastery* in the primary *occupational environment* and *role*?

Occupational Adaptation Programming

What combination of occupational readiness and occupational activity is needed to promote the patient's *occupational adaptation process*?

What help will the patient need to assess *occupational responses* and use the results to affect the *occupational adaptation process*?

What is the best method to engage the patient in the occupational adaptation program?

Evaluation of the Occupational Adaptation Process

How is the program affecting the patient's *occupational adaptation process*?

- Which *energy level* is used most often (*primary* or *secondary*)?
- What *adaptive response mode* is used most often (*pre-existing, modified,* or *new*)?
- What is the most common *adaptive response behavior* (*primitive, transitional,* or *mature*)?

What outcomes does the patient show that reflect change in the *occupational adaptation process*?

- Self-initiated adaptations?
- Enhanced *relative mastery*?
- Generalization to novel activities?

What program changes are needed to provide maximum opportunity for *occupational adaptation* to occur?

Note: the italicized terms are constructs in the occupational adaptation frame of reference.

Reprinted with permission from Schultz, S. & Schkade, J. (1992). Occupational adaptation: Toward a holistic approach for contemporary practice, part 2. *Am J Occup Ther, 46*(10), 925. © the American Occupational Therapy Association, Inc.

that it is absent in the client. Your conclusion is that you have not identified the occupational role and goal that will allow this desire to be demonstrated. Therefore, you continue to seek a client-relevant goal in consultation and collaboration with the client and/or family.

3. Occupational adaptation intervention requires a holistic perspective of the client and all person systems are inevitably present in every occupational response. This is true regardless of the setting in which you practice.

The plan for this book is to lead you through the process and use actual case studies to illustrate the use of occupational adaptation in practice. As the concept is introduced, a case will be offered that emphasizes that particular concept. You will recognize many of concepts other than the one that is featured. This approach will be used to facilitate understanding of the major concepts and how they can be used in practice. We will not attempt to tell you what to "do" as intervention. Occupational adaptation is a way of thinking about intervention from a client-centered, occupation-focused perspective. If you examine Table 1-2, the *Occupational Adaptation Guide to Practice* from Schultz & Schkade (1992), you will notice that it is a series of questions, not a list of prescriptions. The *Guide to Practice* tells you what questions to ask if you want to practice from an occupational adaptation perspective. The answers to those questions guide your interaction with the client, as together you develop a plan for occupational intervention.

The reading list that follows this chapter includes brief annotations that we hope will be helpful to you if you wish to explore occupational adaptation more thoroughly. Mostly, we hope that you will find this book a useful tool for an intervention that we believe will maximize the contribution of both client and therapist to a satisfying outcome that is client-centered and occupationally focused.

REFERENCES

Schkade, J. K. & Schultz, S. (1992). Occupational adaptation: Toward a holistic approach to contemporary practice, Part 1. *Am J Occup Ther, 46*, 829-837.

Schultz, S. & Schkade, J. K. (1992). Occupational adaptation: Toward a holistic approach to contemporary practice, Part 2. *Am J Occup Ther, 46*, 917-926.

OCCUPATIONAL ADAPTATION READING LIST

Buddenberg, L. A. & Schkade, J. K. (1998). A comparison of occupational therapy intervention approaches for older patients after hip fracture. *Topics in Geriatric Rehabilitation,13*(4), 52-68.

Clinical study demonstrating the importance of personally chosen activity.

Crist, P., Royeen, C., & Schkade, J. K. (2000). *Infusing occupation into practice.* (2nd Ed.). Bethesda, MD: AOTA.

This is a transcription of a workshop given by the theorists contrasting occupational adaptation, model of human occupation, and occupational science using a mental health case example. Sally Schultz presents the occupational adaptation perspective.

Dolecheck, J. R. & Schkade, J. K. (1999). Effects on dynamic standing endurance when persons with CVA perform personally meaningful activities rather than non-meaningful tasks. *Occupational Therapy Journal of Research, 19*(1), 40-53.

The patient case that inspired this study appears in the Christiansen & Baum book cited below as Schultz & Schkade, 1997. It's a wonderful case!

Ford, K. (1995). Occupational adaptation in home health: A therapist's viewpoint. *Home Health and Community Special Interest Section Newsletter, 2*(1), 2-4.

Excellent, easy-to-read article.

Garbarini, J. & Pearlman, V. (1998). Fieldwork in home health care: A model for practice. *Education Special Interest Section Quarterly, 8*(4), 1-4.

Excellent use of occupational adaptation to guide student practice in home health.

Garrett, S. & Schkade, J. K. (1995). The occupational adaptation model of professional development as applied to level II fieldwork in occupational therapy. *Am J Occup Ther, 49*, 119-126.

Good explanation of the adaptive response behaviors.

Gibson, J. & Schkade, J. K. (1997). Effects of occupational adaptation treatment with CVA. *Am J Occup Ther, 51*, 523-529.

Clinical study demonstrating functional outcomes.

Jackson, J. P. & Schkade, J. K. (In press). Occupational adaptation model vs. biomechanical/rehabilitation models in the treatment of patients with hip fractures. *Am J Occup Ther.*

Clinical study comparing two intervention approaches with results on functional outcomes and client satisfaction.

Johnson, J. P. & Schkade, J. K. (2001). Effects of occupation-based intervention on mobility in CVA. *Journal of Applied Gerontology, 20*(1), 91-111.

Three cases of home health intervention. Excellent application examples.

Macrae, A., Falk-Dessler, J., Juline, D., Padilla, R., & Schultz, S. (1998). Occupational therapy models. In A. Macrae & E. Cara (Eds.), *Psychosocial occupational therapy, a clinical practice* (pp. 97-125). Albany, NY: Delmar Publishers.
Describes the use of occupational adaptation in mental health practice.

Pasek, P. B. & Schkade, J. K. (1996). Effects of a skiing experience on adolescents with limb deficiencies: An occupational adaptation perspective. *Am J Occup Ther, 50,* 24-31.
Focuses on the relative mastery construct.

Ross, M. M. (1994, August 11). Applying theory to practice. *OT Week,* 16-17.
Nice case written by a therapist who is an excellent practitioner of occupational adaptation.

Schkade, J. K. & Schultz, S. (1992). Occupational adaptation: Toward a holistic approach to contemporary practice, Part 1. *Am J Occup Ther, 46,* 829-837.
Original article, part 1.

Schkade, J. K. & Schultz, S. (1993). Occupational adaptation: An integrative frame of reference. In H. Hopkins & H. Smith (Eds.), *Willard & Spackman's occupational therapy* (8th Ed.). Philadelphia, PA: J. B. Lippincott Co.
Brief description. A longer one is necessary for real understanding.

Schkade, J. K. & Schultz, S. (1993). Occupational adaptation: An example of theory and contemporary practice integration. AOTA, Commission on Education, Short Papers. Abstract.

Schkade, J. K. & Schultz, S. (1998). Occupational adaptation: An integrative frame of reference. In M. E. Neistadt & E. B. Crepeau (Eds.), *Willard & Spackman's occupational therapy* (9th Ed.). Philadelphia, PA: J. B. Lippincott Co.
Another short description. Included with MOHO and Ecology of Human Performance as theories based on occupational behavior.

Schkade, J. K. (1999). Student to practitioner: The adaptive transition. *Innovations in Occupational Therapy Education,* 147-156.
Application to professional transitions.

Schroeder-Smith, K., Tischenkel, C., DeLange, L., & Lou, J. Q. (In press). Duchenne muscular dystrophy in females: A rare genetic disorder and occupational therapy perspective. *Occupational Therapy in Health Care.*
Case study describes impact of a genetic disorder on occupation. Occupational adaptation is used to guide the process of occupational therapy.

Schultz, S. & Schkade, J. K. (1992). Occupational adaptation: Toward a holistic approach to contemporary practice, Part 2. *Am J Occup Ther, 46,* 917-926.
Original article, part 2.

Schultz, S. & Schkade, J. K. (1994). Home health care: A window of opportunity to synthesize practice. *Home & Community Health, Special Interest Section Newsletter, American Occupational Therapy Association,* 1(3), 1-4.

> Good article for understanding the basic approach to intervention. We highly recommend this as a first article to read.

Schultz, S. & Schkade, J. K. (1997). Adaptation. In C. Christiansen & C. Baum (Eds.), *Occupational therapy: enabling function and well-being* (2nd Ed.). Thorofare, NJ: SLACK Incorporated.

> Extensive treatment of the concept of adaptation as a paradigm with a couple of cases using occupational adaptation. Good articulation of the theory. Includes most up-to-date definitions.

Werner, E. (2000). Families, children with autism and everyday occupations. Unpublished doctoral dissertation. Nova Southeastern University, Ft. Lauderdale, FL.

> Innovative use of occupational adaptation with families.

Other Recommended Reading

On Challenge
Csikszentmihalyi, M. (1990). *Flow.* New York: Harper Collins Publishers.

On Transition
Dr. Seuss. (1990). *Oh the places you'll go.* New York: Random House.

On a Balanced Lifestyle: Implications for Adaptation Energy
McGee-Cooper, A. (1992). *You don't have to go home from work exhausted!* New York: Bantam Books.

On Adaptation
Johnson, S. (1998). *Who moved my cheese?* New York: G. P. Putnam's Sons.

CHAPTER TWO

How Do the Person and Environment Relate

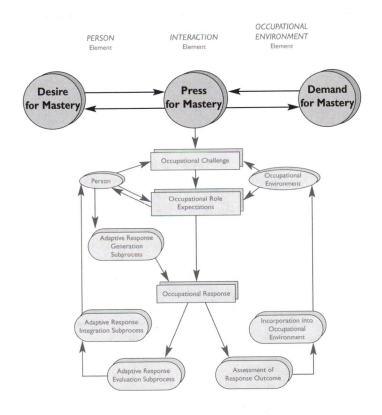

PERSON
Element

INTERACTION
Element

OCCUPATIONAL
ENVIRONMENT
Element

Desire
for Mastery

Press
for Mastery

Demand
for Mastery

Occupational Challenge

Person

Occupational
Environment

Occupational Role
Expectations

Adaptive Response
Generation
Subprocess

Occupational Response

Adaptive Response
Integration Subprocess

Incorporation into
Occupational
Environment

Adaptive Response
Evaluation Subprocess

Assessment of
Response Outcome

CHAPTER CONCEPTS

Desire for mastery, demand for mastery, and press for mastery.

DESIRE FOR MASTERY, DEMAND FOR MASTERY, AND PRESS FOR MASTERY

As seen in the basic process figure (see Figure 1-1), the individual desires to behave masterfully and the environment demands mastery of the person. The interaction of these two influences results in a press for mastery. The *desire for mastery*, the *demand for mastery*, and the *press for mastery* are present throughout life. The desire and demand for mastery produce a dynamic tension between the individual, desiring to confront challenges adaptively and masterfully, and the environment, demanding that the individual respond adaptively and masterfully. At times, individuals effect an interaction that is adaptive and masterful. At other times they do not. Competence in this important interaction is a function of the health and strength of the occupational adaptation process as it develops over time, beginning with birth. Competence can be viewed as relative influence over the person-environment interaction outcomes.

Development of Mastery

The *desire for mastery* exists in a rudimentary form at birth. As the infant experiences some degree of perceived mastery (which emerges serendipitously from random and reflexive action), the repertoire of adaptive occupational responses begins to accumulate and the occupational adaptation process starts to develop.

Development of *desire for mastery* begins with the early need for nurture as the infant is challenged with the necessity of locating the nipple, which she must find in order to receive nutrition. At first reflexive, the nutrition-seeking approach becomes adapted over time to be less reflexive and more intentional.

If you observe the developing toddler at play you will conclude that her *desire for mastery* is obvious as she attempts to be successful at reaching her desired goals. She behaves with a response apparently designed to achieve the goal of reaching a desired object, gathering it closer to her body, producing some change in the object such as separation, attachment, or controlling of parts, etc. Adaptations of posture, movement, effort, and focus can be seen as she attempts to achieve goals. Her desire to master these challenges is obvious even to the casual observer. She is seeking to express her influence over the environment.

The facilitators or barriers that the environment contributes affect expression of the *desire for mastery*. The environment shapes the *demand for mastery* through these barriers or facilitators. For example, a child placed in a playpen is expected to keep explorations within the parameters of the playpen. A child placed on the floor is freer to explore the wider parameters of the room or the house. As the child grows and develops, family expectations for independence or dependence are expressed. Within certain family or ethnic contexts, dependence on others is encouraged; while within other contexts, the family evidently wishes increasing independence on the child's part. The child's *desire for mastery* and the environment's *demand for mastery* are sometimes consonant, sometimes dissonant. The developing child, desiring to experience mastery and increase his relative influence over interactions with the environment, must find an adaptation that allows him to satisfy his own needs for mastery while also satisfying the contextually specific environmental expectations. The interaction of these two demands becomes the *press for mastery*.

Press for Mastery Over the Life Span

The *press for mastery* continues over a lifetime. Factors over which we wish to exert influence change over time. Environmental demands also change, but the need to respond adaptively and masterfully continues. Occupational challenges occur in different locations and contexts, but they do not go away. An important thing to remember is that we move in and out of occupational performance situations where we feel competent. Even very competent people can feel unsure when confronted with significant challenges. Nevertheless, the *press for mastery* exists with interaction from both the person and the environment.

Take the example of the secretary who has been working for 30 years. She is extremely competent with an electric typewriter. She types rapidly and accurately. She knows what the typewriter can and cannot do. She knows how to operate it in a way to obtain the result she desires. She takes pride in her high-quality work (*desire for mastery*). Suddenly, she must produce excellent work with use of a word processor. The employer wants her to continue producing high-quality documents with the same speed and accuracy (*demand for mastery*). The resulting *press for mastery* means that she must now deal with computer hard drives that lose documents that she has input, systems that freeze up and have to be rebooted, work stoppages because electronic systems are inoperative, and other experiences familiar to all who have been confronted with electronic dominance in document production. The important assumption for occupational adaptation is that the *desire for mastery*, the *demand for mastery*, and the *press for mastery* are constants in the area of competence in occupational functioning even when circumstances change.

Organizational or process changes in work situations are everywhere. Reorganization, downsizing, managed care, and reimbursement changes in health care are powerful examples that therapists encounter on an almost daily basis. The dynamic tension between the personal professional desires of the therapist and the health care system can intensify. Nevertheless, the therapist wishes to respond adaptively and masterfully for the benefit of her clients and the security of her job. The employer expects that the therapist will respond adaptively and masterfully for the benefit of clients and the organization. The best-selling book *Who Moved My Cheese?* (Johnson, 1998) tells a very engaging and thought-provoking story of the tension between the person and the occupational environment. It illustrates the interaction of the two under changing conditions. It provides examples of what happens to mastery when the individual either pays attention to or tries to ignore environmental demands in his quest to preserve his *desire for mastery*.

It is very easy for therapists to assume that clients no longer have a desire for mastery. The case of the Afghan Maker (see next page) illustrates what a therapeutic error such an assumption can be.

THE AFGHAN MAKER

The following case is a result of two occupational therapy students serving a client in a nursing home during their senior year. Their clinical reasoning and theoretical considerations are reflected in summary after class treatment team discussions.

Mrs. Turner is an 84-year-old woman living in a nursing home. Her medical chart indicated that she had been discharged on two previous occasions from occupational therapy services secondary to refusal to participate in prescribed activities.

The students assumed before seeing Mrs. Turner that she did not have a *desire for mastery* due to her limited participation in activities listed in her chart and her documented decline in cognitive status.

During the initial session, occupational therapy students assessed Mrs. Turner's interests. She had minimal interests in the present; however, she did voice a strong participation in the past with crocheting. Because of Mrs. Turner's limited stated interests and history of depression, the students reasoned that their client was isolating herself in her room and would benefit from leaving her room to participate in other home activities. Mrs. Turner adamantly refused to leave her room despite the student therapists' rationales and explanations. The occupational therapy students further reasoned that because their client did not want to leave her room and she was requiring assistance in ADLs as documented by nursing staff, she would have the desire to work on increasing her independence in ADLs. This idea was declined by Mrs. Turner. The students then attempted several cognitive activities designed to address Mrs. Turner's deficits in memory and orientation. Although these activities involved current events and card games, Mrs. Turner demonstrated marginal engagement and limited attention span. The students finally reasoned that Mrs. Turner's past interests were the way to go. They left a ball of light blue yarn and crochet hook with her at the end of their session with the hopes of enticing interest in their next session. The next week when they returned, Mrs. Turner had not only managed to crochet a circular medallion with the light blue yarn, she had managed to secure multiple colors of yarn and showed off a crocheted mini afghan! Mrs. Turner was able to demonstrate the various stitch patterns to the students, as well as tell the students her plan of getting yellow yarn to finish it off.

This case demonstrates that the students' assumption that Mrs. Turner did not have a *desire for mastery* was false. The implications for practice are that a therapist must always assume that a *desire for mastery* is present. The occupational therapist must explore possibilities until the client's *desire for mastery* is identified.

Case reported by: Stephanie Springfield, OTS
Nanette Tabani, OTS

REFERENCE

Johnson, S. (1998). *Who moved my cheese?* New York: G. P. Putnam's Sons.

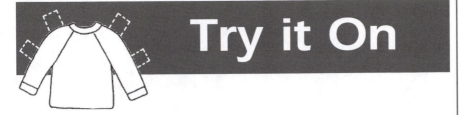

Try it On

Now that we've laid some of the foundational concepts, it is time to "try it on" yourself. We will ask you to think about this example throughout the book as the occupational adaptation process unfolds. To begin, identify an event in your life that produced a need for you to behave adaptively and affected your ability to function adaptively. Maybe your event occurred at work as you transitioned into a new position, or purchased a new home, or adjusted to your favorite leisure activity following an injury or age-related changes. As you contemplate your life event, think about how your desire for mastery and the environment's demand for mastery occurred.

Life event:_____

Person	Environment
Why did you desire to have mastery in this situation?	How did the environment make its demands known?

CHAPTER THREE

How Do Occupational Role Expectations Fit in

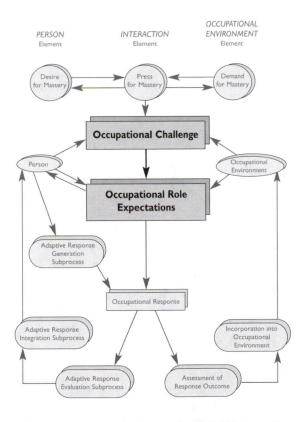

CHAPTER CONCEPTS

Occupational challenge, internal and external expectations,
person and occupational environment.

The press for mastery described in Chapter Two takes the form of an *occupational challenge* in particular situations. The *occupational challenge* may range from one that is fairly minor in scope and temporary in duration to one that is major in scope and of extended duration. The *occupational challenge* emerges from occupational roles and the interaction of expectations associated with those roles. Therefore, *occupational role expectations* are central to occupational adaptation. **It is the *occupational role expectations* that produce the need for the occupational adaptation process to go to work.**

Occupational role expectations have two sources: person-generated expectations (internal) and environment-generated expectations (external). To understand how occupational adaptation interprets these expectations, we have to take a look at how the frame of reference views the person and the environment (Figure 3-1).

The Occupational Environment and External Expectations

The *occupational environment* is the context in which a particular occupational role is carried out. There are many ways to think about this context. Occupational adaptation proposes to think about it as *work, leisure/play,* or *self-care occupational environments.* These are very familiar ideas in occupational therapy and ones that come naturally to occupational therapists. While *occupational environments* in general can be categorized this way, the specific features of a particular *occupational environment* are different from another one within the same category. For example, your work circumstance may be very different from that of a professional friend even though you are both occupational therapists. What creates the differences is that each has influences that make each work environment what it is. Occupational adaptation labels these influences as *physical, social,* and *cultural subsystems.* In other words, the *physical, social,* and *cultural subsystems* represent the nonhuman and human factors within a work setting. The same thing can be said of leisure *occupational environments* as well as self-care *occupational environments.*

The subsystems in a particular *occupational environment* supply the *external occupational role expectations.* For example, suppose one of your favorite leisure occupations is attending professional baseball games. The way in which you carry out your role as a spectator will be influenced by the physical features of the parking lot, the stadium, the seats, locations of restrooms and concession stands, etc. (the *physical subsystem*). Friends or family who attend the game with you, people seated around you, and those who stand in line with you form the *social subsystem.* If you are a

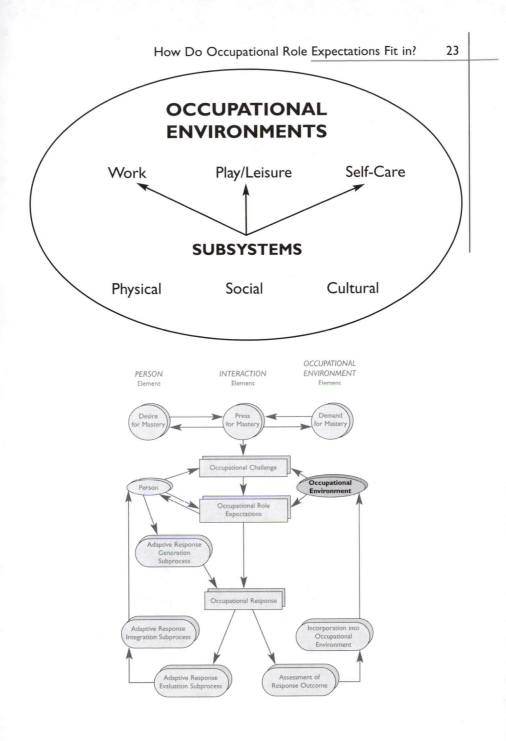

Figure 3-1. Occupational environments and subsystems.

parent accompanying children, the social expectations will be different than on occasions when you are attending the game with adults only. The *cultural subsystem* consists of all the customs, rules and regulations, mission, or purpose. For example, the seventh-inning stretch is a part of the *cultural subsystem*, as is cheering for the home team and playing the National Anthem to begin the event.

These *physical, social,* and *cultural subsystems* tell us what the *external role expectations* are in a particular situation. The specifics will differ as the *occupational environments* differ, but the same principle applies (Figure 3-2).

The Person and Internal Expectations

In addition to the external expectations, the individual brings his or her own set of internal expectations to any *occupational challenge*. So, how does occupational adaptation view the individual? Once again, familiar occupational therapy ideas are used. In occupational adaptation, the person consists of three systems: *sensorimotor, cognitive,* and *psychosocial systems*. Just as each *occupational environment* has unique features because of physical, social, and cultural influences, so each individual has unique sensorimotor, cognitive, and psychosocial capabilities because of *genetic, environmental,* and *experiential/phenomenological subsystems* feeding into them. Genetic and familial factors can have a powerful influence on the individual's internal role expectations. For example, tasks that favor having a certain physiological feature, such as a small body and a well-coordinated sensorimotor system, will not result in very positive internal role expectations if the body is large and poorly coordinated. Likewise, one's current or enduring environmental circumstances can predispose the individual to certain internal expectations. If a task requires economic or social resources that are unavailable, expectations will be colored by that situation. Similarly, the individual's history or experience adds a phenomenological quality to the picture. If the experiences have been positive, the expectations are more positive. If experiences have been negative, the expectations will likely be more negative. All these influences will impact our assessment of the likely outcomes and therefore give rise to a unique set of *internal role expectations* when confronting an *occupational challenge*.

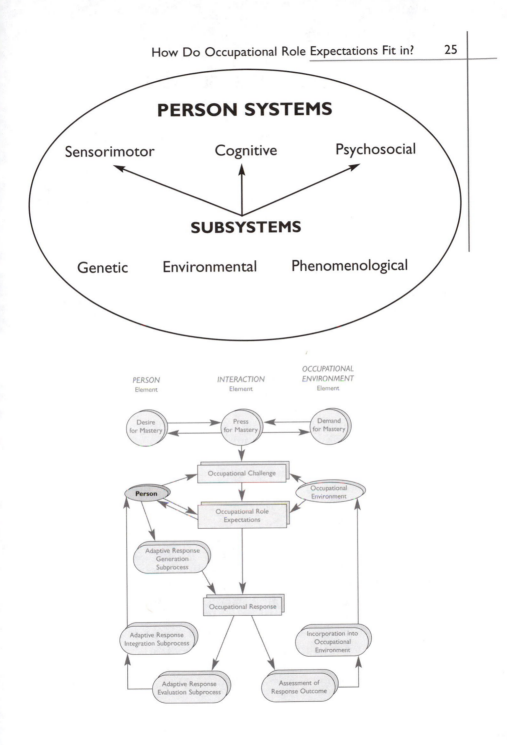

Figure 3-2. Person systems and subsystems.

Occupational Challenge and Interacting Expectations

The *occupational challenges* presented to the individual are thus embedded within roles having expectations that are idiosyncratic to the individual performing within a particular environmental context. For example, while there are common attributes within the parent role (i.e., care for the survival and developmental needs of one's children), there are substantial differences that stem from the physical, social, and cultural demands of the specific *occupational environment* in which the parental role encounters a challenge. A parent responding to the behavior of a child who has violated a rule of the household is in a very different position from the parent who responds to a teacher's request for a conference based on that same child's failure to perform satisfactorily in the school environment. Both of these situations involve the parent role, but the environmental contexts within which these challenges must be confronted are distinctively different.

For the therapist, the importance of role expectations is that they become the structure upon which you plan and implement intervention with the collaboration of the client. The client and/or family will have to help you understand those expectations, particularly if it is a role with which you are unfamiliar or whose expectations are very different environmentally from your own knowledge and experience. Therapist understanding of the expectations is important whether your focus is on an individual who is experiencing those minor/temporary challenges expected as a part of living, or one with major but temporarily disruptive challenges, or one with chronic disabling conditions that result in major and persistent challenges.

The therapist must not assume that he or she knows the *occupational role expectations* for a particular client. In many cases, the client becomes the teacher and the therapist the learner. This relationship sets the stage for a true collaboration between client and therapist. The client brings his or her knowledge of the expectations and the therapist brings his or her expertise in occupational functioning. See the case of the Water Skier on the next page. The Water Skier demonstrates how attention to the occupational role demands as the client experiences them can lead to a very effective and satisfying outcome for all concerned. It also empowers the client to be an active and collaborative participant in the therapy process.

THE WATER SKIER

Mr. Moore was a 27-year-old single male who was referred to a hand clinic for therapy following surgery for a flexor tendon laceration of the left wrist. Return to work was the original focus of the OT intervention. However, Mr. Moore's disinterest in therapy led the therapist to consider other occupational roles as more important to the client. She learned that what motivated him was the opportunity to return to competitive water skiing, an occupational role that was very important to him.

Since the therapist knew nothing of the demands of this occupational role, the client had to educate her about the requirements of competitive water skiing. First, he taught her about the physical demands of this environment. She learned that the demands included static and dynamic handling of equipment with speed and accuracy, maximum resistance to the upper extremities, and good overall body condition. It also required grasping and manipulating a ski rope handle. It required ability to comfortably maintain a stable grasp with moderate to maximum force. It also required the ability to rapidly manipulate the handle between hands. Endurance and strength to resist force of the water and the rope were also required.

The client also taught her about the social aspects—interaction with competitors, team members, and officials. The cultural demands included performance according to competition regulations—speed, time, and number of tricks performed. Learning about the occupational role performance demands led to a collaborative intervention plan that was focused on gradually preparing Mr. Moore to return to the occupational role demands of competitive water skiing. The therapist included tissue-healing goals. She also included graded functional activities to improve object manipulation and progression to simulation of ski rope handle manipulation with progressive resistance. Return to water skiing competition began with engagement in the social expectations, progressing to driving the boat for other skiers.

Through focus on an occupational role and its demands that were personally meaningful to the client, an intervention plan was developed in which the client was actively and enthusiastically engaged. This approach led to a very therapeutic outcome. The surgeon's and the therapist's tissue healing goals were met. The client's occupational goals were met.

Case reported by Kimberly Norton, MS, OTR/L, CHT in Schultz, S. & Schkade, J. K. (1997). Adaptation. In C. Christiansen & C. Baum (Eds.), *Occupational therapy: enabling function and well-being* (2nd Ed., pp. 478-479). Thorofare, NJ: SLACK Incorporated.

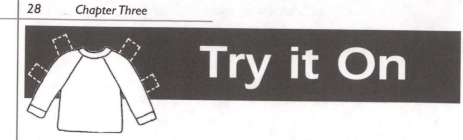

Now we will take the life event that you identified in the last chapter as providing a need for adaptation. What were the role expectations you had for yourself that made this situation an occupational challenge? What were the role expectations from the environment that contributed to the occupational challenge? Remember the occupational challenge is a function that you need or want to carry out. Also remember these role expectations are intimately related to your desire for mastery and the environment's demand for mastery.

Occupational challenge: _____

You: Internal Role Expectations	Environment: External Role Expectations
What did you expect of yourself in this role and the challenge it presented?	What did the environment expect of you in this role and the challenge it presented?

In the next chapter, we will ask you to continue reflecting on these expectations as we explore the internal process of how persons respond to challenges and try to meet those expectations.

CHAPTER FOUR

How Does the Person Begin to Produce the Response

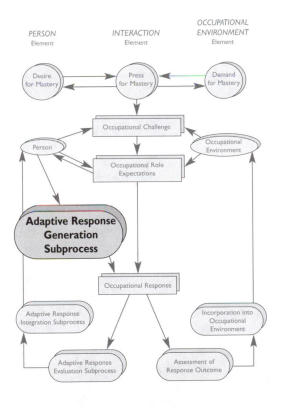

PERSON
Element

INTERACTION
Element

OCCUPATIONAL
ENVIRONMENT
Element

Desire for Mastery

Press for Mastery

Demand for Mastery

Occupational Challenge

Person

Occupational Environment

Occupational Role Expectations

Adaptive Response Generation Subprocess

Occupational Response

Adaptive Response Integration Subprocess

Incorporation into Occupational Environment

Adaptive Response Evaluation Subprocess

Assessment of Response Outcome

CHAPTER CONCEPT

The adaptive response generation subprocess (adaptive response mechanism).

The person has a perception of the role expectations within a particular occupational challenge. The next steps are to create a response, evaluate it, and integrate it. These steps occur through the action of subprocesses within the individual's occupational adaptation process. These subprocesses are known respectively as the *adaptive response generation subprocess*, the *adaptive response evaluation subprocess*, and the *adaptive response integration subprocess*. The function of the subprocesses is to facilitate an adaptive response, hence their name. They do not always produce an adaptive response, just as a dysfunctional cardiovascular system may not pump blood to the extremities in a satisfactory manner. Nevertheless, the function for which the cardiovascular system exists does not change and we do not change the name. Neither do we rename an *adaptive response subprocess* that is dysfunctional. Each of these subprocesses exists to facilitate adaptive responses to challenges. When there is dysfunction in one or more of these subprocesses, the occupational adaptation process is dysfunctional.

The first subprocess is the one where the response gets created. The creation of the response is the work of the *adaptive response generation subprocess*. The next two chapters will be devoted to the *adaptive response generation subprocess*. This is an abstract idea but a very important one. It is also the most unique feature of occupational adaptation and probably its greatest contribution to occupational therapy intervention. Therefore, it is important to roll up your sleeves and wrestle with these ideas in order to master them. In short, this is where the real fun begins.

THE ADAPTIVE RESPONSE GENERATION SUBPROCESS

The *adaptive response generation subprocess* is the anticipatory portion of the occupational adaptation process. From a therapeutic perspective, this anticipatory activity is where the OT intervention will need to have its ultimate impact. In other words, as a therapist you desire that the client will be able to anticipate the outcomes of self-generated responses. Anticipating potential outcomes, both good and bad, promotes more adaptive and masterful responses.

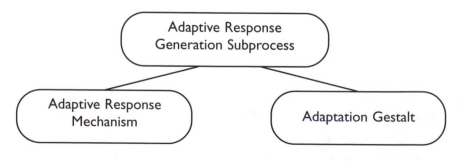

The *adaptive response generation subprocess* consists of two components: the *adaptive response mechanism* and the *adaptation gestalt*. The *adaptive response mechanism* does some preliminary work in generating the response, and the *adaptation gestalt* plans the holistic inclusion of sensorimotor, cognitive, and psychosocial systems. This chapter will focus on the *adaptive response mechanism*. Chapter Five will deal with the *adaptation gestalt* component.

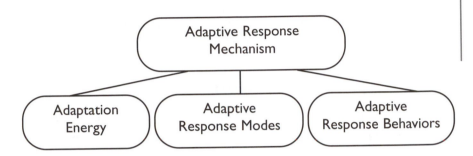

Adaptive Response Mechanism

The response creation flow begins when the individual activates the *adaptive response mechanism*. Within the *adaptive response mechanism* is the energy that drives the process (*adaptation energy*), the patterns of responding to challenges that have developed with time and experience (*adaptive response modes*), and the particular behavior types or classes that the person uses in an attempt to respond adaptively (*adaptive response behaviors*). Table 4-1 lays out the components and principal characteristics of the *adaptive response mechanism*. All three components of the *adaptive response mechanism* are active simultaneously. There is no particular order in which these components act, nor is one more significant or important than the other. Do not think of them as a hierarchy. We are simply "freeze-framing" the process, once again, in order to understand how the *adaptive response mechanism* operates.

Adaptation Energy

The person systems (sensorimotor, cognitive, and psychosocial) are capable of energizing the adaptation process at two levels of awareness simultaneously. Selye's notion (1956) of *adaptation energy* has influenced the perspective of occupational adaptation. Selye's scientific work was on the impact of stress on the adrenal glands, as seen in laboratory animals. He went on to generalize about the human condition with thought-provoking logic based on his animal findings. While Selye has influenced the thinking about adaptation energy in occupational adaptation, the concept is understood and used very differently.

Table 4-1

ADAPTIVE RESPONSE MECHANISM

Adaptation Energy	Adaptive Response Modes	Adaptive Response Behaviors
Primary: Focused attention; high energy usage at intense activity; more structured *Secondary:* More creative, sophisticated; low energy usage; disregards structure in favor of alternative approaches	*Existing:* Response patterns in adaptive repertoire from previous successful uses *Modified:* Changes in existing mode when existing mode fails to achieve success *New:* Uniquely different mode developed as existing and modified fail to achieve success	*Primitive:* Hyperstabilized in all person systems; "frozen" or stereotypic; no adaptive movement (no variety in behavior that can lead to adaptation) *Transitional:* Hypermobile in all person systems; high activity level; random; unmodulated; variable Variability can result in behavior more likely to produce response that can lead to adaptation *Mature:* Blended mobility and stability in all person systems; goal-directed; modulated; most likely to produce adaptive and masterful response to challenge

Reprinted with permission from Schultz, S. & Schkade, J. K. (1997). Adaptation. In C. Christiansen & C. Baum (Eds.), *Occupational therapy: enabling function and well-being* (2nd Ed., p. 476). Thorofare, NJ: SLACK Incorporated.

Adaptation energy is the "fuel" that drives the occupational adaptation process. Occupational adaptation views *adaptation energy* as being bounded (finite), after the assumption of Selye. It is important not to confuse "finite" with "small." The notion of an energy that is bounded calls for efficient use of that bounded supply so that it can last a lifetime for adaptive needs.

Therapists frequently object to the notion of *adaptation energy* being bounded. However, there are other parallels to a finite supply in nature. For example, it is thought that we are born with all the neurons we will ever have. Barring disease, trauma, or abuse, this is a supply to last a lifetime. It is also thought that female infants are born with all the ova they will ever have. This, too, is enough to last a lifetime. Why does occupational adaptation take the view that *adaptation energy* is bounded? If we assume that energy does have limits, then it is important to manage it wisely so that it can last a lifetime. Occupational adaptation proposes that the way to maximize benefits and increase longevity of the supply of *adaptation energy* is to utilize its two levels—primary and secondary—in such a way as to produce the most efficient, effective, and satisfying outcomes.

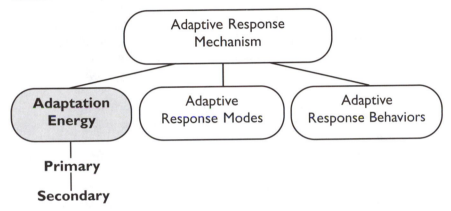

Primary adaptation energy is active when there is intentional and focused attention directed to the occupational challenge at hand. *Secondary adaptation energy* is active when intentional and focused attention is directed away from the occupational challenge at hand. As can be seen in Table 4-1, *primary adaptation energy* uses adaptation energy at a faster rate, particularly when the activity is focused at a high intensity. Lower intensity focus at the primary level uses less adaptation energy. *Secondary adaptation energy* acts at a lower awareness level than does *primary adaptation energy* and uses energy at an even slower rate.

How does energy use and occupational challenge response relate? When we approach problem solution at the primary level, we tend to set up problem-solving structures. This can be a good strategy. However, these structures can actually limit creative problem solving when we let them restrict us to the boundaries of a particular structure. We often have to work harder (use more primary energy) when we try to force solutions within boundaries. More creative and sophisticated *secondary adaptation energy* goes beyond the problem solution boundaries we set up when primary energy is active. It turns our boundaries upside down and all around, and disregards their limits. Use of *secondary adaptation energy* leads to those sudden, creative, and insightful solutions. Because it is assumed to use less adaptation energy, *secondary adaptation energy* is therefore more efficient. It is logical, then, that use of increased secondary energy is an effective tool in managing a bounded supply of energy.

When you alternate between primary energy and secondary energy you are most likely to experience the most efficient, effective, and satisfying use of the limited supply. **The occupational challenge must initially be worked on at a primary level.** The desired result is that the problem is then shifted or "shunted" to the secondary energy. This shift of focus takes place either after primary energy activity fails to reach a solution, or the demands of life send you to the grocery store or your child's soccer game. The problem is then shunted to secondary energy for further activity while the primary energy becomes directed to another task. This is somewhat similar to the multitasking computer environments that allow multiple projects to be worked on in parallel for greater efficiency (i.e., one program is running in the foreground while another is running in the background). For the multitasking environment to work each of the programs must be loaded, an activity similar to working first at a primary energy level.

As an example, an occupational therapist who was one of our students was working on an important term project. This project was worth a significant percentage of the course grade. She had thought about the project a great deal. Every approach she considered seemed to lead to a deadend (primary energy). Although she was skeptical about the effectiveness of the occupational adaptation principle of shunting her project to secondary energy, she decided to leave the project and knit a sweater for the infant she was expecting in a few weeks. When she completed the sweater, she returned to her project, and the elements of the project and the approach she needed to use were clear to her. In other words, secondary energy working on her course project while primary energy worked on knitting a sweater was a more efficient way to reach her goal of developing the course project. All she had to do was execute the solution in written form.

This therapist/student would normally have completed her project at a primary energy level. She would have doggedly stayed on task until it was completed and expended a great deal of primary energy in the process. She would have spent more total time developing her product and bringing it to a completed written form than she did with knitting a sweater at the same time she conceptualized her project.

The construct of adaptation energy allows for an explanation of why occupation-focused intervention works to promote positive outcomes for clients we serve. Engagement in activity at a primary energy level directed away from attention to person system deficits allows activity at the secondary energy level to produce solutions. Thus, intervention that allows patient responses to emerge more "automatically" (less studied and focused effort) is more likely to produce the desired therapeutic outcome. See the case of the Preacher on the next page, based on Dolecheck and Schkade (1999) and Schultz and Schkade (1997). The Preacher illustrates how a change in the therapist's approach resulted in the client's ability to use secondary energy to enhance functioning of a dysfunctional sensorimotor system while primary energy was focused on a personally meaningful occupational activity.

Adaptive Response Modes

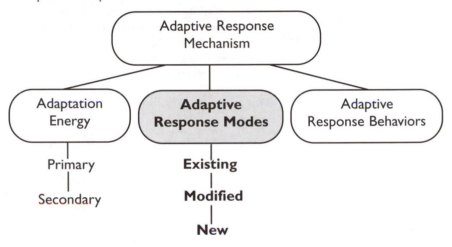

Adaptive response modes are another feature of the *adaptive response mechanism*. Patterns of responding to occupational challenges that have resulted in at least some degree of mastery become incorporated into the individual's adaptive response repertoire as *adaptive response modes*. *Adaptive response modes* are classified as *existing adaptive response modes* (those already in our repertoire), *modified adaptive response modes* (those in which we make changes in an existing mode), and *new adaptive response modes* (those that come about because our existing or modified modes are not working for a particular need).

Adaptive response modes begin to develop as the infant behaves reflexively and randomly. These reflexive and random movements sometimes produce unintentional effects on persons and objects. For example, an infant is lying in supine kicking his legs as part of the natural development of sensorimotor capability. Quite by accident, he kicks a bell that is

THE PREACHER

Mr. Jones was a 68-year-old African-American retired minister who had suffered a stroke. He presented with the characteristic neurologic damage that left him with problems in movement and speech. His multidisciplinary rehabilitation team had been concentrating intervention on the *sensorimotor system* (i.e., emphasis on standing tolerance, shifting his weight while standing, being able to reach across his body in diagonal patterns, speech articulation disorders). After considerable time and effort, the team had concluded that the patient was not a good candidate for walking. His documented standing tolerance was a maximum of 5 minutes and his difficulty in weight shifting was extreme.

At this point, the therapist was introduced to occupational adaptation and the importance of focusing intervention on personally meaningful activity. In a conversation with Mr. Jones, the therapist discovered that he was a preacher and most desired to return to that *occupational role*. She told him that the next day she would bring a podium into the room where the Bible study group, of which Mr. Jones was a member, would meet and she wanted him to preach. Mr. Jones expressed fear and apprehension that he would not be able to preach. The next day, a Friday, the therapist brought a podium into the room and put it in place. As soon as Mr. Jones saw this symbol of the *physical subsystem* from the *occupational environment* of preaching, he began to articulate a list of things he could talk about. Despite his apprehensions about standing and talking, Mr. Jones was assisted into standing and began to preach. For 20 minutes, Mr. Jones stood and preached. As he preached, he weight-shifted. He gestured, crossing midline, to the full extent of his range of motion. He spoke in the most powerful voice he could summon. At the end of the 20 minutes when Mr. Jones sat down, he burst into a song. Then he cried. The following Monday, Mr. Jones began to walk. By engaging Mr. Jones in the activity of preaching, the sensorimotor and speech deficits were shunted to *secondary adaptation energy* while primary energy was focused on the activity of preaching. As the sensorimotor and speech requirements were shunted to the *secondary energy* for assistance, the capabilities of the sensorimotor system had been "unbound" from the structure imposed by standard protocol clinical intervention at the primary energy level. Engagement in an *occupational activity* that was meaningful to Mr. Jones based on the role expectations associated with preaching set the stage for him to maximize remaining capabilities and act as his own agent of therapeutic change. The sensorimotor and speech performance requirements were thus allowed to emerge in a more automatic fashion.

Case reported by Jessica Dolecheck, MA, L/OTR

suspended above his crib. As he repeats the kicking movement and continues to experience the bell sound, he begins to make associations between these actions and certain outcomes. This it the manner in which the *adaptive response modes* that produce particular outcomes become a part of the collection of familiar response patterns.

When confronted with an occupational challenge, ordinarily our first attempt is to use existing modes. They have worked in the past and "why reinvent the wheel?" When an existing mode produces some degree of mastery, it is more efficient to use that mode, as you have to expend effort and *adaptation energy* to develop a new one. If, however, the use of an existing mode does not produce some degree of mastery, there is a reason to explore an alternate method. In the example of the infant kicking the bell, he may use the kicking movement in an attempt to produce some other outcome. Kicking may not have the desired effect and thus lead the infant to explore other response modes. Sometimes a slight modification of an existing mode will produce the desired result. It is a reasonable approach to simply "tweak" an already comfortable approach (a modified mode). At other times, even a substantial modification of an existing mode will not produce a satisfactory outcome. On these occasions, there is the impetus to create an entirely new pattern of interaction in order for an *adaptive response* to be realized (a new mode). See the case of the Researcher on the next page. The Researcher illustrates how an occupational challenge can require the development of a new *adaptive response mode* and how the therapist facilitates the development of the new mode.

Remember that *adaptive response modes* are patterns of responding to environmental cues that the individual develops. Frequently, the therapist must assist a client to develop either modified or new *adaptive response modes*. Current capabilities may not allow use of existing *adaptive response modes*.

Adaptive Response Behaviors

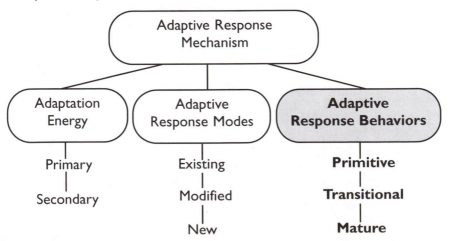

THE RESEARCHER

Dr. Smith was a 33-year-old physician from Ghana, Africa who had come to the United States to study for a PhD in anatomy. As the result of an automobile accident, his nondominant left arm had to be amputated at the shoulder. His greatest concern was that he would be unable to complete the research for his dissertation, which involved the study of human brain tissue. After learning from Dr. Smith what the *external* and *internal role expectations* were, the therapist, in collaboration with Dr. Smith, developed a plan of intervention. They concluded that the most pressing need was to be able to continue the tasks associated with data collection, analysis and written reporting. To engage in the tasks of his chosen *role*, it was essential that Dr. Smith develop new or modified *adaptive response modes* using one-handed approaches to respond to his *occupational challenges* until a prosthesis could be fitted and training in its use carried out.

As part of his occupational adaptation intervention program, the therapist included *occupational readiness* goals such as increase in right upper extremity endurance, increased knowledge of assistive equipment and one-handed techniques, and fluidotherapy for pain in the right hand. His *occupational activities* included discussion and demonstration of his ability to carry out functions in his research laboratory (i.e., operation of a cryostat and ultramicrotome using a diamond cutter on a pyramid base [approximately 1-inch square] to prepare very thin slices of tissue samples for examination under a microscope, and placing and removing samples from the microscope). Dr. Smith and the therapist made a trip to his laboratory to problem-solve ways in which he could use one hand. Because Dr. Smith was also interested in ADL and IADL activities, the intervention plan included his one-handed construction and use of an assistive fingernail clipper and file board; ADL skills in dressing with assistive devices or one-handed techniques; driver re-education with the use of a spinner knob for steering, stopping/parking, and advancing; community activity including filling a car with gasoline, transferring from car to ground, selecting food from a buffet, eating independently, asking for help when entering/exiting doors, and carrying a plate back to the table.

On a return trip to the clinic following discharge, Dr. Smith reported to the therapist that he had installed a turning knob on the steering wheel of his car to allow him to drive with one hand. Dr. Smith's

continued on next page

The Researcher, continued

pre-accident existing *adaptive response mode* of using two hands could not successfully be used until his prosthesis was ready and he had been trained in its use. He had to develop a new one-handed mode, which he used successfully. Thus, the therapist assisted Dr. Smith in developing a new *adaptive response mode*. In the future when the prosthesis becomes a part of his functional picture, he will have to modify his previous two-handed mode to accommodate to the prosthesis. He will likely continue use of his new one-handed mode for certain tasks if he experiences the prosthesis to be cumbersome.

Case reported by DeLana Honaker, PhD, OTR

Adaptive response behaviors are the third feature of the *adaptive response mechanism*. *Adaptive response behaviors* are types of behavior that we use in attempting to respond adaptively and masterfully. Occupational adaptation classifies these behaviors as *primitive, transitional*, and *mature* (see Table 4-1 for characteristics of each). The labels for these behavior classes were inspired by the work of Gilfoyle, Grady, and Moore (1981, 1990) in their articulation of spatiotemporal adaptation. As in the case of the *adaptation energy* construct and the influence of Selye (1956), we have departed substantially from the work of Gilfoyle, Grady, and Moore in our use of these labels. Despite our recasting of these labels to a significant degree, it is appropriate to acknowledge the influence of these theorists in labeling these behaviors. Gilfoyle, Grady, and Moore's characterization of primitive, transitional, and mature behaviors is part of a developmental scheme to describe sensorimotor development in the infant and young child. In normal sensorimotor development, the child progresses from primitive to transitional to mature sensorimotor behaviors. While in occupational adaptation the classes of behavior do develop with experience in responding to naturally occurring challenges, the development of mature behaviors does not preclude the use of primitive and transitional behaviors over the course of normal occupational functioning. Each of these classes of behavior remains in our behavioral repertoire. We use each class at various times under certain conditions. These behavior classes are not considered hierarchical, but simply different forms of behaving. See Table 4-1 for examples of how the classes of behaviors might present in the three person systems.

Primitive Adaptive Response Behaviors

Primitive adaptive response behaviors are those that individuals frequently use when experiencing extreme difficulty and stress while attempting to respond adaptively and masterfully to occupational challenges. *Primitive behaviors* are characterized as *hyperstable* in that they present as a kind of "stuckness." They occur in all three person systems. It is important to recognize primitive behaviors as "normal" when the individual feels overwhelmed by a particular challenge. Thus, their occurrence should be expected and not considered dysfunctional when they are used as a temporary balance-restoring attempt. When they are used for a protracted period, adaptive movement is prevented.

Transitional Adaptive Response Behaviors

Transitional adaptive response behaviors, in contrast to the primitive behaviors, are characterized by *hypermobility*. Instead of the invariance and immobility of the primitive behaviors, the *transitional behaviors* are highly variable, not well modulated, very active, often random, and without clear goal direction. Like the primitive behaviors, they occur in all three person systems. *Transitional behaviors* may follow primitive behaviors when the individual becomes "unstuck" but is still unable to arrive at a problem solution. The *transitional behaviors*, however, do provide variability in solution attempts, some of which may provide adaptive movement and in some cases even provide a solution. They frequently function as an intermediate step between hyperstable behaviors and mature ones, although this is not always the case.

Mature Adaptive Response Behaviors

Mature adaptive response behaviors are those exemplified by a *blended mobility/stability* in all the person systems. Behaviors are modulated, goal directed, logical or insightful, and solution oriented. It is important to remember that *mature behaviors* may not be the first behaviors seen in an attempt to respond adaptively and masterfully. The individual may use primitive and transitional behaviors, perhaps moving in and out of those classes before arriving at the *mature behaviors*. When the individual uses *mature behaviors* to find a truly adaptive response to one challenge, there is no assurance that *mature behaviors* will be used at the onset of a new challenge. All three classes of behavior remain in our adaptive response behavior repertoire. En route to an adaptive solution, we may use all three classes at various times in situations where the challenge is complex and multifaceted. Thus, emergence of these classes of behavior is to be expected and not a cause for discouragement. Only if no adaptation develops after a reasonable period of time are primitive and transitional variations considered dysadaptive.

The case of the Chess Player, Mr. Barnes, exhibits how the therapist facilitates adaptive movement through the classes of adaptive response behaviors. It is also an outstanding example of a therapist approaching treatment holistically. Instead of ignoring the patient's psychosocial dysfunction, she attended to it therapeutically and effectively, thereby achieving the desired goals associated with his physical dysfunction.

THE CHESS PLAYER

Mr. Barnes was a 58-year-old male hospitalized for a total hip replacement and accompanying rehabilitation. He also had a history of depression and presented with many behaviors consistent with obsessive compulsive disorder. He was well known for his chess-playing skill, as evidenced by his picture on the cover of a chess magazine. Mr. Barnes was extremely anxious and had difficulty focusing on therapy because of anxieties regarding such things as cleanliness, bowel movements, staff who were uncooperative to his many demands, medical bills, etc.

In occupational therapy sessions, Mr. Barnes focused on complaints and anxieties, which his therapist and psychologist believed were more related to his fears regarding loss of control and death. In accordance with the physician's referral and the protocol for rehabilitation following total hip replacement, the therapist focused on educating Mr. Barnes about hip precautions. However, his anxieties interfered with his compliance with hip precautions. Mr. Barnes was hyperstable in his focus on anxiety and despair.

The therapist discussed with Mr. Barnes his feeling of loss of control and the behaviors he had that acted this out. Together they looked at the positive and negative aspects of these behaviors and how they affected his performance and satisfaction in daily life. They spent some time on relaxation techniques to help him get "unstuck" from his hyperstability. They agreed that he would make a list of his concerns before the occupational therapy sessions. He and the therapist then discussed the list and which concerns he could do something about, what his options were, and what things he could let go of. The psychologist helped to educate the staff regarding obsessive compulsive disorder and how they might better interact with Mr. Barnes.

Mr. Barnes responded to the plan and began to perform ADLs in a way that was somewhat satisfying to him. However, he was impulsive and had to receive constant cuing by the therapist to pay atten-

continued on next page

The Chess Player, continued

tion to hip precautions and safety (his hyperstability had been replaced by hypermobility). The therapist pointed out that attention to detail and the ability to remember rules was what made him successful in playing chess. She recommended that he use this same approach in remembering and executing the hip precaution "rules."

His impulsivity in ADLs began to decrease and he prided himself on remembering the hip precaution "rules." He still required occasional cuing in novel situations to comply with the precautions. His interaction with staff improved for those staff members who were able to give Mr. Barnes choices. At discharge 2 weeks later, he was functioning at moderate independence in ADLs. He demonstrated his ability to generalize hip precautions and safety to novel activities. His basic obsessive approach still pervaded his life, but he did occasionally initiate relaxation techniques. His list of concerns in the hospital became minimal and he began to realistically assess his options to those concerns without assistance (Mr. Barnes was demonstrating behavior that was an adaptive blend of mobility and stability).

Case submitted by Joanna Lipoma, MOT, OTR

The occupational adaptation process is at its most obvious during times of life transitions that impact occupational functioning. These transitions may be normative, such as a transition from spouse to parent, student to professional, staff member to manager, etc. During major life transitions (exemplified by the transition from functioning as an able-bodied young adult to a young adult with a spinal cord injury), the adaptation process is most at risk for disruption. A premorbid adaptation process that is functioning marginally will be most vulnerable and the impact of a dysfunctional process the most profound. The well-functioning adaptation process will be less vulnerable but will be challenged to the limits of its intact and healthy operation. During these life transitions, the various classes of the adaptive response behaviors—primitive, transitional, and mature—will be most evident.

The *adaptive response mechanism* is obviously a very abstract description of how the adaptive response begins to develop. Two occupational therapists who specialize in the practice of hand dysfunction created a model of how you might see the *adaptive response mechanism* in a client. These two therapists reflected on the responses they had seen in their clients and found striking examples of how their clients demonstrated the aspects of this mechanism. This model (see grey box on next page) pro-

ADAPTIVE RESPONSE MECHANISM MODEL

Adaptation Energy

Primary: Learning exercise and use of splints and equipment.
Secondary: Exercises and positioning incorporated into a daily routine, position or dynamic devices during sleep, reintegration of the hand into self-maintenance, work, or leisure activities.

Adaptive Response Modes

Existing: Use of currently available coping skills, cognitive skills, problem-solving approaches.
Modified: Enhancement of coping skills and ownership, enhanced self-discipline for adherence to the program, change routine to allow for treatment time.
New: Development of new coping skills, own the injury and recovery process, structure time or gain outside support to make time and energy available for treatment.

Adaptive Response Behaviors

Primitive (hyperstabilized): Fear of ownership, fear of reinjury, fear or unwillingness to return to previous tasks or roles. Example: the dependent patient; the patient sees the role as "victim of accident or treatment process"; he or she may be a submissive participant in a structured treatment plan.
Transitional (hypermobile): Preoccupation with details of the treatment program, search for more "things" that will help, search for advice from anyone and everyone. Example: the patient brings in popular media reports of unusual or novel treatments.
Mature (blended mobility/stability): Sees the injury as an event to be dealt with, takes initiative in treatment planning and implementation. Example: active participant in a cooperatively designed treatment process.

Model contributed by: Gail Blom, MA, OTR, CHT
Kim Norton, MA, LOTR, CHT

vides a good summary of the *adaptive response mechanism* in practice. It demonstrates responses that clients frequently exhibit as they progress through the challenges accompanying the need for adaptation following injury, trauma, or illness.

SUMMARY

To this point we have talked about how occupational adaptation views the person and the occupational environment. We have addressed the occupational challenge and role expectations from both the person and the occupational environment. Once the person encounters an occupational challenge and begins to develop a response, the adaptive response mechanism comes into play. The adaptive response mechanism is part of the internal process that occurs as a person develops a response to an occupational challenge. The components of this internal mechanism have been examined in this chapter and illustrated by therapist-reported cases. The second part of the adaptive response mechanism is the *adaptation gestalt*, which is the topic of the next chapter. The adaptation gestalt describes how the person involves sensorimotor, cognitive, and psychosocial features in the upcoming response.

REFERENCES

Dolecheck, J. R. & Schkade, J. K. (1999). Effects on dynamic standing endurance when persons with CVA perform personally meaningful activities rather than non-meaningful tasks. *Occupational Therapy Journal of Research, 19*(1), 40-53.

Gilfoyle, E., Grady, A., & Moore, J. (1981). *Children adapt.* Thorofare, NJ: SLACK Incorporated.

Gilfoyle, E., Grady, A., & Moore, J. (1990). *Children adapt.* (2nd Ed.). Thorofare, NJ: SLACK Incorporated.

Schultz, S. & Schkade, J. K. (1997). Adaptation. In C. Christiansen & C. Baum (Eds.), *Occupational therapy: enabling function and well-being* (2nd Ed.). Thorofare, NJ: SLACK Incorporated.

Selye, H. (1956). *The stress of life.* New York: McGraw-Hill.

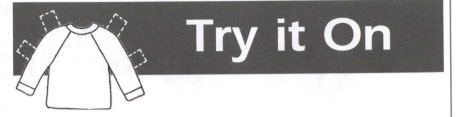

Try it On

Now this is where the fun begins... We will ask you to reflect on how you went about preparing to respond to your occupational challenge. The following tables will help lead you through the process.

Occupational challenge (from Chapter Three): _____

ADAPTIVE RESPONSE GENERATION SUBPROCESS

Adaptation Energy	Adaptive Response Modes	Adaptive Response Behaviors
Primary Secondary	Existing Modified New	Primitive Transitional Mature

Let's enlarge each of these components for a closer look. Remember we are continuing to focus on your identified occupational challenge.

Adaptation Energy	Yes/No
Primary? While engaged in responding to your particular challenge, did you find yourself initially focused with high energy and high concentration to your task and remain there for the duration of the activity?	
Secondary? While engaged in responding to your particular challenge, did you find yourself at first highly focused and concentrating on your task, then leaving it for a time to do something else? Did you then return to your task and find you had made progress on a problem solution even while actively doing something else?	

Further observations:

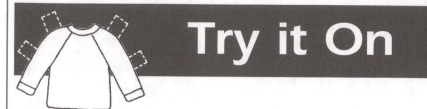

Try it On

Adaptive Response Modes	Yes/No
Existing? Did you find that you were engaged with your challenge the same way that you always have? Routine? "Same old, same old?"	
Modified? Did you find that you were engaged with your challenge in some ways the same, but you tried something different? "Living slightly on the edge?"	
New? Did you find that you approached your challenge with a whole different approach? "Life in the fast lane?"	

Other thoughts:

Adaptive Response Behaviors	Yes/No
Primitive? Did you find that when you were engaged in responding to your challenge, you were just plain stuck (hyperstable)?	
Transitional? Did you find that when you were engaged in responding to your challenge, you were moving fast and in no apparent planned and organized direction (hypermobile)?	
Mature? Did you find that when you were engaged in responding to your challenge, you experienced thoughtful problem solving and adaptation based on a combination of reason and creativity (blended mobility and stability)?	

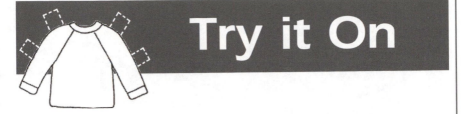

When you were preparing your responses, did you find yourself "bouncing around" among these three types of behavior? If you did, that's okay. Remember these are simply classes of behavior, all of which exist to help with an adaptive response.

Additional reflections:

In the occupational adaptation process, these components (adaptation energy, adaptive response modes, and adaptive response behaviors) are dynamic actions, flowing naturally in the context of the challenge. In the next chapter we will examine the gestalt or plan of action.

CHAPTER FIVE

What's the Plan to Carry Out the Response

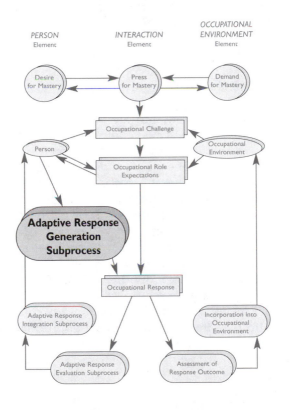

PERSON
Element

INTERACTION
Element

OCCUPATIONAL
ENVIRONMENT
Element

Desire
for Mastery

Press
for Mastery

Demand
for Mastery

Occupational Challenge

Person

Occupational
Environment

Occupational Role
Expectations

**Adaptive Response
Generation
Subprocess**

Occupational Response

Adaptive Response
Integration Subprocess

Incorporation into
Occupational
Environment

Adaptive Response
Evaluation Subprocess

Assessment of
Response Outcome

CHAPTER CONCEPT

The adaptive response generation subprocess (adaptation gestalt).

The remaining component of the adaptive response generation sub-process (where the occupational response gets created) is the *adaptation gestalt*. The *adaptation gestalt* takes the work of the adaptive response mechanism (adaptation energy, adaptive response modes, and adaptive response behaviors described in Chapter Four) and produces a plan for the response.

THE ADAPTATION GESTALT

An important assumption of occupational adaptation is that every person system (sensorimotor, cognitive, and psychosocial) is present in every response. The three person systems then must be configured into a plan for the occupational response. This plan is called the *adaptation gestalt*. Since a gestalt is a type of image in which the whole is greater than the sum of its parts, the gestalt label seems appropriate for the plan that occupational adaptation is describing. The *adaptation gestalt* is a way to think about holistic responding and intervention.

Each person system is not necessarily present to the same degree in every *adaptation gestalt*. Different tasks require different plans. If a task is essentially cognitive, then the cognitive person system should be dominant, the sensorimotor system should be operating to provide movement or nonmovement appropriately, and the psychosocial system should be operating to provide an adaptive level of motivation while keeping factors such as anxiety from interfering with performance. A student taking an examination probably needs the plan just described (Figure 5-1).

Suppose, however, that the student is competing in a gymnastics event. Now the task is predominantly sensorimotor. In this instance, the sensorimotor system should be dominant; the cognitive system should be sufficiently involved to provide memory of the rules of competition that can affect performance, as well as movements and their sequence; and the psychosocial system is involved so as to provide an adaptive level of arousal and motivation for that individual (Figure 5-2).

When the task is primarily psychosocial, as in comforting a friend who has lost a family member, the psychosocial system must be at its most sensitive and effective, the cognitive system appropriately involved to assist with solution identification, and the sensorimotor system permitting whatever activity that will allow the friend to carry out the comforting function adaptively (Figure 5-3).

In other words, the *adaptation gestalt* balance will differ from one situation to another if adaptive occupational functioning is to be realized. **There is no one "balanced" *adaptation gestalt* that fits all persons and situations.** It is highly idiosyncratic to the situation and to the individual. It is easier to think about the *adaptation gestalt* with a visual representa-

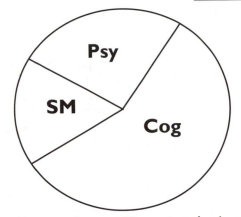

Figure 5-1. Adaptation gestalt—cognitive system dominant.

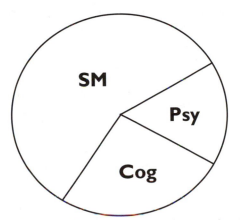

Figure 5-2. Adaptation gestalt—sensorimotor system dominant.

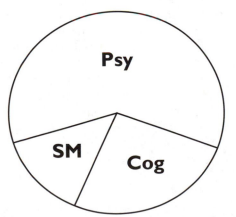

Figure 5-3. Adaptation gestalt—psychosocial system dominant.

tion. A simple circle divided into parts to represent the relative presence of each person system is helpful.

It is important for therapeutic intervention to recognize that all three person systems are present in each occupational response. When the occupational adaptation process has been made dysfunctional because of trauma, disease, chronic conditions, etc., that process cannot be improved without attention to all three person systems regardless of the nature of the disabling condition. For example, if an individual is so depressed after suffering a stroke that she has no desire to participate in rehabilitation, the therapist will be hard pressed to achieve any therapeutic results in sensorimotor and cognitive systems while the psychosocial system is dominating the *adaptation gestalt*. If the therapist can facilitate a change in the *adaptation gestalt* so as to bring the person systems into a better balance for the task of rehabilitation, the impact of therapy will be much more effective in addressing the patient's occupational adaptation process. All concerned should experience a better outcome. Focusing on an occupation that is important to the client is the optimal way to facilitate an *adaptation gestalt* configuration that is most likely to produce an improvement in occupational functioning. See the case of the Husband Caregiver. The Husband Caregiver illustrates how the therapist facilitated a rebalancing of the *adaptation gestalt* to produce a therapeutic outcome based on the demands of the client's primary occupational role.

THE HUSBAND CAREGIVER

Mr. Brown was an 82-year-old male who was hospitalized following a stroke. His previous medical history included hypertension and prostate cancer. His wife of 54 years was expected to live no more than 6 months because of terminal lung cancer. A number of years earlier she had been diagnosed with breast cancer, which was followed by a mastectomy. She had never regained full range of motion or strength in the affected extremity. As a result of Mrs. Brown's problems, Mr. Brown had been assisting her with upper extremity dressing, self-care, and cooking for many years. In the initial assessment, when the therapist asked Mr. Brown about his primary occupational interest, he indicated that it was to do everything he could to help his wife in the ways to which they had become accustomed (i.e, his caregiving role). Assessment of the person systems revealed:

- Sensorimotor system: Active range of motion in the left extremity to be within functional limits with muscle strength and grip strength rated as a 3+ out of 5, limited range of motion in the

continued on next page

The Husband Caregiver, continued

right extremity with muscle and grip strength rated as a 2+ out of 5. Bilaterally, his sensation (light touch, pain, stereognosis, kinesthesia, proprioception, and temperature) was within functional limits. He required minimum assistance in bed mobility. His static sitting balance was rated as good, while his dynamic sitting balance was rated a fair+. His endurance was sufficient to tolerate sitting on the side of the bed with minimum fatigue during an evaluation that lasted approximately 45 minutes. Mr. Brown reported to the therapist that he was trying to perform simple hygiene and sponge bathing with one hand.

- Cognitive system: The therapist found that Mr. Brown was oriented to person, place, and date. His attention span and concentration during the evaluation were within functional limits and his perception was to be evaluated during activities of daily living.
- Psychosocial system: Assessment revealed a husband who was depressed and tearful as he discussed with the therapist his wife's impending death. He expressed guilt that his prostate cancer had been healed while his wife's cancer had not. He voiced strong desire to concentrate only on spending time with his wife. He was not interested in therapy for himself. Assessment of Mr. Brown's occupational environment yielded information that the couple lived in a two-bedroom home with assistive bathroom equipment, which included a tub transfer bench, elevated toilet seat, and hand-held shower. The Browns lived in a neighborhood where the neighbors were supportive.

Mr. Brown's *occupational role* of caregiver became the basis for intervention. It was clear to the therapist that Mr. Brown's *adaptation gestalt* was extremely dominated by a *psychosocial system* that was depressed and grieving, making it difficult to engage the *sensorimotor* and *cognitive systems*, which were the reasons for the occupational therapy referral. Her task was to develop an intervention that would facilitate the reconfiguration of Mr. Brown's *adaptation gestalt* to reflect the importance of the *psychosocial system* at this time in his life, while also allowing the *sensorimotor* and *cognitive systems* to become more active.

The therapist devised all aspects of the intervention plan with Mr. Brown's preferred occupational role of caregiver directing her thinking. She developed *occupational readiness* interventions (interventions in the person systems to help prepare them for the occupation

continued on next page

The Husband Caregiver, continued

of caregiver). These interventions included minimal resistance Theraband activities and balloon batting activities with his wife, wrist weights added as tolerated, medium resistance and hand putty exercise, proprioceptive neuromuscular facilitation trunk stabilization exercise, and simple hygiene and hemi-dressing techniques for himself. *Occupational activities* (intervention in which the client was actively engaged in his chosen occupational role) included assisting his wife with upper extremity dressing by using assistive equipment (to address endurance, dynamic sitting balance, trunk stabilization, upper extremity strength, grip strength, hemi-dressing technique, and motor planning in the *sensorimotor* and *psychosocial systems*); assisting her with simple hygiene by using his affected right arm as a stabilizing unit (to address weight-bearing, proprioception, balance, and upper extremity strength in the *sensorimotor, cognitive,* and *psychosocial systems*); working with her to put together a photo album (to address the *cognitive system* as stories were retold with dates/places/people, *sensorimotor system* with grip strength and endurance, and *psychosocial system* with the grief process); cooking easy breakfasts/lunches/dinners with her (to address *cognitive, sensorimotor,* and *psychosocial systems*).

Based on Ross (1994)

The *adaptation gestalt* is a simple, straightforward way to conceptualize how an individual "plans" an occupational response. This way of creating an image of one's response may be useful in assisting individuals to anticipate the outcome of their occupational response before the response has been acted out and thus provide one way to self-correct dysfunctional responses.

REFERENCE

Ross M. M. (1994, August 11). Applying theory to practice. *OT Week*, 16-17.

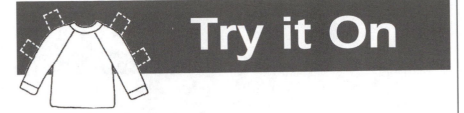

ADAPTATION GESTALT

Don't let the word *gestalt* deter you. This concept, as stated before, is simply your "plan of action." For example, an occupational therapy student enters her first patient's room on internship with the task to begin an initial assessment. She finds herself so nervous and anxious she cannot think about how to begin the assessment. Her mind is inundated by the multitudes of assessments she has learned in school as she mentally scans through them with the hope that the right one will soon surface. She thinks about how disappointed her clinical instructor will be when she finds that the assessment hasn't progressed. She widens her base of support, grasps her clipboard tightly, and tries to ignore her shaking knees. Been there? The following depicts how this student's gestalt may have looked. Notice that while her psychosocial system predominates, her cognitive and sensorimotor components are still present.

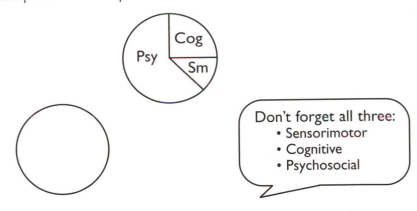

Don't forget all three:
• Sensorimotor
• Cognitive
• Psychosocial

Now it's your turn. The occupational challenge that you identified in Chapter Three is still the "work in progress." Take a look at your "plan of action" in how you generated your response. Using the circle as a pie, separate out the person divisions and their involvement with your challenge.

Any reflective thoughts?

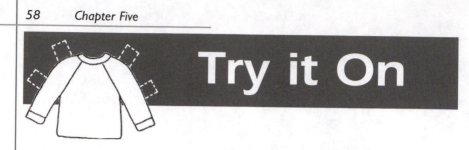

OK, you've finally responded to the challenge at hand. The next chapter will explain how persons go about evaluating the outcome of their attempts to respond adaptively and masterfully. This will involve discussion of the next subprocess of the system: the adaptive response evaluation subprocess.

CHAPTER SIX

What's Right or Wrong With This Picture

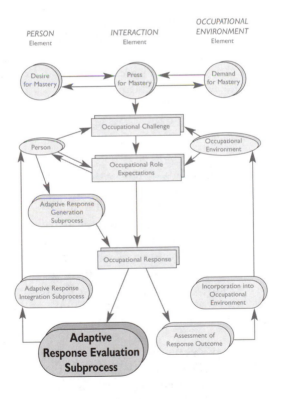

The adaptive response evaluation subprocess (relative mastery).

ADAPTIVE RESPONSE EVALUATION SUBPROCESS

After the occupational response has been carried out, the next important step is for the individual to evaluate the outcome produced by the response. This evaluation takes place through the action of the *adaptive response evaluation subprocess*. For adaptation to occur, we have to evaluate our occupational responses. Otherwise, we continue to repeat previous responses whether or not they were useful in achieving the goal for which they were intended. **In other words, the leading edge of adaptation is awareness that the response needs to change for some perceived reason.**

The self-evaluation subprocess begins with *activation* of the evaluation function. This activation step involves a "what's right with this picture or what's wrong with this picture?" question to initiate evaluation. Occupational adaptation proposes that the core action of the subprocess is a phenomenological assessment tool called the experience of *relative mastery*. The word *phenomenological* emphasizes that *relative mastery* is an individualistic experience. Is *relative mastery* the same thing as skill mastery? Definitely not! We want to be clear about that. Do not confuse *relative mastery* with skill mastery that is evaluated by an external source with external criteria to guide the evaluation.

Relative mastery consists of three properties:
1. Efficiency (use of time, energy, and resources)
2. Effectiveness (the extent to which the response achieved the desired goal)
3. Satisfaction to self/society (the extent to which the person experiences satisfaction with the outcome, and the extent to which relevant society feels satisfied with the outcome)

Let's take an example of a professional tennis player to illustrate the difference between *relative mastery* and skill mastery. Suppose we have a world-class tennis player. On one week he is playing in a major tournament where he is the top seed (officials who run the tournament expect him to win the tournament). He makes it to the final match where he loses in three sets (the worst possible outcome). As he evaluates his performance in the tennis tournament, his self-assessment might look like this:

- Efficiency: Since the match was relatively short, he used less time, energy, and personal resources than he would have if the match had been longer. Therefore, his efficiency was relatively high.
- Effectiveness: Definitely not effective since he did not win.
- Satisfaction to self/society: Very unsatisfying to the player and not satisfying to his fans, who wanted him to win. Satisfying to those who wanted his opponent to win.

Suppose the next week the same tennis player is again playing in a major tournament. This time he wins in a grueling five-set match. He might evaluate his *relative mastery* like this:

- Efficiency: Not efficient, because it was a long match that took a great deal of time, energy, and personal resources.
- Effectiveness: Very effective since he won.
- Satisfaction to self/society: A very satisfying outcome. It is satisfying to win in a long, demanding match. Tennis-watching society also likes a five-set, demanding match.

The important point to be made here is that the skill mastery of the tennis player was the same over the 2 weeks. Yet, his experience of *relative mastery* changed markedly from one week to the next.

In similar fashion, the client with whom the therapist is intervening may have criteria that are important to him that do not show up on the therapist's assessment as an external evaluator. The therapist is likely using various assessment tools such as standardized, norm-referenced, or functional independence evaluations. Those externally determined evaluations are of merit for documentation and/or reimbursement purposes; however, from the standpoint of occupational adaptation, these evaluations are used in conjunction with the client's self-assessment of *relative mastery*. The client has a perspective of his or her internal expectation and those of a specific environment on which intervention is focused. For example, the therapist may evaluate a skill competence level as low because of movement substitution patterns that deviate from some established norm. **A client, however, may view a personal response as being reasonably efficient, very effective, and highly satisfying to self and society because the response is carried out in a manner that is consonant with internal expectations and/or physical, social, and cultural expectations of the relevant occupational environment.** For example, therapists frequently report anecdotally that clients abandon assistive devices when they are discharged because they find other ways of doing things that are more personally satisfying.

One important thing to remember from a therapeutic standpoint is that you are attempting to intervene in the client's internal adaptation process. Giving the client an opportunity to assess his or her own progress in terms of experience of *relative mastery* provides the client with a tool for evaluating occupational responses after the therapy is over and the client returns home.

Because *relative mastery* is idiosyncratic to the individual, that individual determines what constitutes the extent to which he or she has experienced efficiency, effectiveness, and satisfaction to self/society. That individual takes into account the occupational role demands (internal and external) for the activity in question and reaches a personal conclusion about the individual experience of *relative mastery*. As an overall assessment of the occupational event (the plan for the response, the response itself, and the outcome), the individual is thought to place the event somewhere on a conceptual continuum between occupational adaptation and occupational dysadaptation with homeostasis as a midpoint. In other words, from awareness of the challenge, to perception of the internal and external role expectations, to formation of a plan for action, to the outcome and finally its effect on the experience of *relative mastery*, the individual concludes that his or her interaction with the occupational environment was somewhere between a "disaster" and a "triumph." The information gained from this self-assessment indicates to the client whether further adaptation is needed. For an example of how the client's assessment of *relative mastery* can be used therapeutically, see the case of the Florist. The Florist illustrates how the client's assessment of relative mastery led to self-directed changes in his intervention plan.

THE FLORIST

Mr. Green was a 54-year-old engineer who had sustained a bilateral cardiovascular accident (CVA). When first seen by the therapist he was comatose and initially unable to engage actively in his intervention. Working closely with Mrs. Green, the therapist learned that Mr. Green enjoyed music and that the Greens owned a flower shop where Mr. Green worked in addition to his job as an engineer. While Mr. Green was comatose, his beginning intervention consisted of *occupational readiness* activities on the part of the therapist and Mrs. Green. The plan consisted of bilateral upper and lower extremity passive range of motion exercises, sitting balance activities, and sensory stimulation. Mr. Green proved to be responsive to vestibular stimulation, slow rocking, icing, and auditory stimulation, such as bells and the therapist singing songs by a popular singer who was known to be liked by Mr. Green. Mrs. Green was given instructions in passive range of motion, and positioning techniques were taught to nursing staff and Mr. Green's family. By week 3, following surgery and medication, Mr. Green made excellent progress and was able to actively engage in his program. Mr. Green indicated tearfully that he wanted to make a special flower arrangement for his wife to celebrate their upcoming anniversary. Thus, his *occupational role* as florist became the guide to intervention, and the therapist was able to place emphasis on *occupational activity* that was relevant to the role of florist.

continued on next page

The Florist, continued

The therapist educated herself by conducting an activity analysis of flower arranging and obtained a supply of silk flowers. She consulted with Mrs. Green as well into the ways in which she and Mr. Green carried out the activities of flower arranging in their florist business.

Mr. Green began planning and making weekly floral arrangements while he was responding and adapting to the changes in his person systems brought on by the CVA. Each week Mr. Green evaluated his progress in *relative mastery* (efficiency, effectiveness, and satisfaction to self/society). As a result of these weekly self-evaluations, Mr. Green made the following adjustments to his intervention plan:

1. For more *efficiency*—during the session prior to the one in which he was to create a flower arrangement, he planned first in his mind and then on paper the particular arrangement he wanted to create.

2. He began taking weekly pictures to see his improvements, which resulted in greater *satisfaction to self*.

3. Mrs. Green began leaving the arrangements he had made at the nurses' station for the weekend to reinforce feelings of *satisfaction to society*.

4. He requested a more rigorous room exercise program to increase his endurance and strength.

5. He borrowed flower books to re-educate himself for an increased feeling of *effectiveness*.

6. Before transfer to a rehabilitation setting, Mr. Green began to help one of the nurses plan the flowers for her wedding.

Case reported by Melissa McClung, MOT, OTR

The goal of including the client in self-evaluation of his progress is two-fold. First, it can assist the client to identify his improvement and his contribution to that improved status. Second, the capacity to evaluate his responses when therapy ends is an empowerment tool that can assist him in all areas of his occupational life to identify when his responses are satisfactory and when they need to be changed. The lack of an ability to evaluate one's responses can result in perseveration of dysadaptive behavior with extended and sometimes very dysfunctional outcomes.

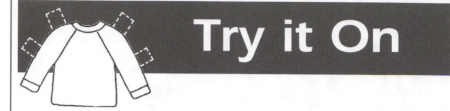

Try it On

Up until now you have been focusing on the generation or creation of your response. Reflect on the response you actually executed. Now it's time for you evaluate that response. *Relative mastery*, a hallmark of occupational adaptation, relates to your perception of how efficient, effective, and satisfying to self and society your response was. Think about your challenge once again, and evaluate your sense of relative mastery.

Relative Mastery	Circle One of the Following in Each Category				
	1 (low)	2	3	4	5 (high)
Efficiency? How efficiently did you use your time, energy, and/or resources while you were engaging in responding to your challenge?	1	2	3	4	5
Effectiveness? To what extent did you accomplish what you set out to do?	1	2	3	4	5
Satisfaction to self and society? How much satisfaction did you experience with your response?	1	2	3	4	5
How about others?	1	2	3	4	5

OK, you've been faced with an occupational challenge. You've generated a plan to meet the challenge and responded. You have evaluated your response. Lastly, you need to focus on how you integrate this occupational event into your overall capacity for adaptation. Chapter Seven will deal with this integration action.

How Has the Person Changed or Adapted

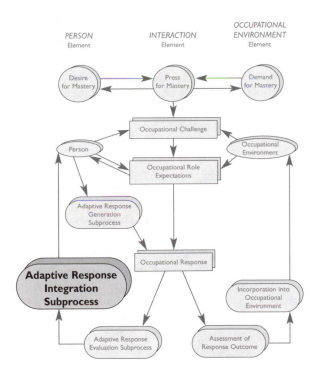

CHAPTER CONCEPT

The adaptive response integration subprocess.

ADAPTIVE RESPONSE INTEGRATION SUBPROCESS

Following activity of the adaptive response evaluation subprocess, synthesis of the occupational event and its integration into the person systems becomes the work of the *adaptive response integration subprocess*. It is in the action of this third subprocess that the adaptation process culminates and impacts the individual's state of occupational functioning as the result of a particular occupational challenge and its subsequent response. In other words, this is where all the information in the occupational event becomes translated and stored into a form that the person can use in the future. Occupational adaptation proposes that one of three states of occupational functioning will be strengthened or reinforced in the person as a result of the adaptive response integration subprocess: *occupational adaptation, homeostasis*, or *occupational dysadaptation*.

A memory of the occupational event that is stored in the person systems activates this process. This memory is an essential precursor to what change or adaptation, if any, develops. In other words, if the individual is to respond to similar challenges in the future, what might that individual do differently to respond more adaptively and masterfully? What did the individual learn about the relationship between the way in which the occupational response was created and the outcome it produced? If the individual's assessment of his or her response was that it did produce a positive experience of relative mastery, then the state of occupational adaptation will be strengthened. Perhaps only minor adjustments in planning similar responses in the future will produce even better results. Perhaps no change is called for. If, as a result of the assessment, the individual found that the experience of relative mastery was more negative than positive, major adjustments may be necessary in the future to produce satisfactory results. If the individual recognizes the dysadaptive nature of the response and still produces no change in the manner in which subsequent and similar challenges are confronted, then the state of occupational dysadaptation will be strengthened or reinforced.

Can a dysadaptive response ever lead to strengthening of the state of occupational adaptation? Indeed it can. Aversive events can be very powerful stimuli for adaptation. When the person, through the action of the adaptive response evaluation subprocess, concludes that he or she does not want to experience the negative relative mastery in the future, significant change can occur. Persons whose occupational adaptation process is dysfunctional may be unable to take advantage of the impetus for adaptation present in events experienced as aversive. It may be necessary for them to continue responding in dysadaptive ways until the adaptive response evaluation and *adaptive response integration subprocesses* can function more successfully. The individual who does not engage the evaluation and integration functions will continue to respond in dysfunctional ways because the necessary functions of these important subprocesses are not operating effectively or, in some cases, not operating at all.

Let's return for a moment to Jill, our new mother in Chapter One. Her initial experience of negative relative mastery did not lead to change even though adaptation was clearly called for. She decided to repeat the same dysfunctional actions. She will simply "try harder." She may have to cycle through the process several times before she reaches an awareness that substantial change is in order. If her occupational adaptation process is functioning well, she will likely be able to make adaptations that will enhance her experience of relative mastery. A very hopeful sign is that she did at least evaluate her response. Her capacity to evaluate appears intact.

When the *adaptive response integration subprocess* is functioning well, adaptation becomes an option for the individual. If the goal of intervention is to intervene in the internal adaptation process of the individual, what are the indicators that this internal process has indeed been impacted?

There are certain indicators that the occupational adaptation process is functioning as the individual confronts and responds to occupational challenges:

1. The client will be experiencing increased relative mastery as he or she responds to occupational challenges.
2. The client will demonstrate spontaneous generalizations to novel tasks without prompting by the therapist or others.
3. The client will initiate adaptations not previously seen or specifically suggested.

All three of these indicators point to internal factors at work. From practice in a home health setting, see the case of the Elder Homemaker. This case illustrates spontaneous generalization and initiation of adaptations. The Elder Homemaker exemplifies indicators of the internal adaptation process at work. The client experienced increasing relative mastery over the course of therapy. As she did so, she upgraded her goals. She also demonstrated spontaneous generalization of skills to tasks and self-initiated adaptations. This case illustrates how the client can direct the course of therapy with the help of a therapist when intervention is focused on occupational activities that are meaningful to the individual.

THE ELDER HOMEMAKER

Mrs. Johnson was a 66-year-old female with uncontrolled diabetes. She had been found unconscious and subsequently hospitalized. Prior to this time, she had become progressively bed-bound and had not walked for the 3 months prior to the hospitalization. In addition to being severely malnourished and debilitated (she weighed less than 80 pounds), she had been consuming a bottle of bourbon every 2 days for some time. She was diagnosed with diabetic ketoacidosis and peripheral neuropathy. She lived alone with her adult son, who was infrequently employed and sometimes undependable. Upon discharge from the hospital, she was referred to a home health agency for occupational therapy.

During the first OT session, an interview was conducted and goals were set. At the next visit, Mrs. Johnson sat at the side of the bed briefly while the therapist explored her interests. Mrs. Johnson indicated that she had been a talented craftswoman but no longer cared to engage in that activity because of failing eyesight and loss of sensation in her fingertips as a result of the peripheral neuropathy. She did agree that at the next session she would sit in a wheelchair and play cards. When, in session three, it was time to transfer to the wheelchair, Mrs. Johnson was apprehensive about the therapist's ability to safely carry out the transfer. The therapist explained the mechanics of the transfer, including the concept of weight-shifting. Mrs. Johnson was able to transfer with minimal assistance and was pleased with how smoothly the transfer was accomplished. She sat in the chair for 1 hour playing cards and expressed pleasure with this accomplishment (increased *relative mastery*).

In session four, Mrs. Johnson transferred with minimal assistance. At her request, the client and therapist moved to the kitchen, which was piled high with dirty dishes and trash. Together they put dishes in the dishwasher and cleaned countertops. Mrs. Johnson volunteered that if her coffee can and filters were placed lower, she could make coffee by herself (*self-initiated adaptation*). In session five, the therapist suggested that they work on transferring from the bed to the bedside commode. Mrs. Johnson informed the therapist that she had already been doing that by herself (*spontaneous generalization*). She also informed the physical therapist that she had stood at the kitchen sink for 3 minutes during occupational therapy. As a result, the physical therapist ordered a walker and gait training progressed rapidly.

continued on next page

The Elder Homemaker, continued

In subsequent sessions, Mrs. Johnson baked corn bread, made soup, and asked to sweep the kitchen floor. Her next goal was to transfer to the bottom of her bathtub. The therapist reported that over the course of intervention there were many updated goals as Mrs. Johnson's confidence grew and her goals became more ambitious. Thus, Mrs. Johnson was directing the course of therapy as a result of her *internal occupational adaptation process* at work. She was evaluating the outcome of her *occupational response* and selecting the next *occupational challenge*.

Based on Ford (1995)

REFERENCE

Ford K. (1995). Occupational adaptation in home health: a therapist's viewpoint. *Home Health & Community Special Interest Section Newsletter, 2*(1), 2-4.

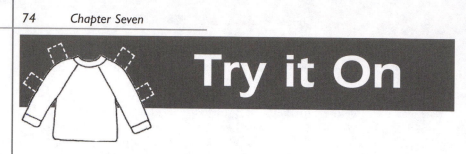

Try it On

You've been quite busy in this section of the book. You've generated a plan for your challenge, responded, and evaluated your response. The following table will guide you toward identifying factors for integration.

Adaptive Integration Subprocess	Comments
Learning: Using your challenge as a base for reflection, think about your expectations, and how your plan and response to your challenge compare. Now reflect upon your sense of relative mastery. What did you learn?	
Modification of the person system: When faced with the same challenge, what would you do differently? Would it be your expectation? (Perhaps how you generated or planned your response.)	

The occupational adaptation process continues, as the environment will be the next focal point.

CHAPTER EIGHT

How Does the Environment Respond

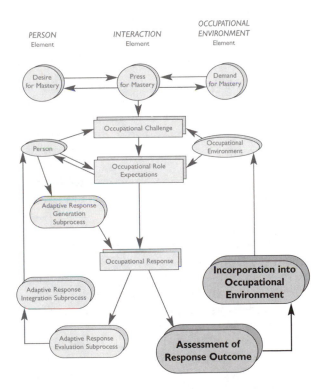

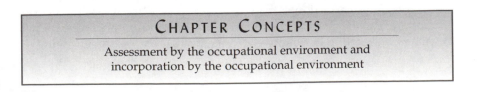

CHAPTER CONCEPTS

Assessment by the occupational environment and
incorporation by the occupational environment

SUMMARY OF THE INTERNAL OCCUPATIONAL ADAPTATION PROCESS

The *internal occupational adaptation process* has been described from the point of view of the individual interacting holistically with the occupational environment through occupational challenges. The person must recognize that a challenge exists and develop a perception of both internal and external role expectations. With this perception to guide the process, the individual generates an occupational response designed to produce an outcome viewed as masterful by both self and society. Upon expression of the response, the individual then evaluates its impact in terms of the extent to which positive or negative relative mastery was experienced. Following evaluation, the individual synthesizes the occupational event, and the results become integrated into the person as learning and adaptation.

EVALUATION BY THE OCCUPATIONAL ENVIRONMENT

The discussion thus far has centered on the individual responding to an occupational challenge. The occupational environment is not idle during this process, but an active participant. The occupational environment contributes substantially to the nature of the occupational challenge and, on occasion, may be the primary determinant of the characteristics in which the challenge appears. It has profound impact on the occupational role expectations since it functions as the source of expectations external to the individual. Through the actions of the physical, social, and cultural subsystems, these external expectations take on shape, texture, and tone. Thus, the influence of the subsystems carries great importance for the individual desiring to respond to the occupational challenge with a response that is adaptive and masterful. Once the occupational response has been expressed, the occupational environment also assesses that response, reflected against the external expectations (i.e., feedback).

There are indicators of physical, social, and cultural subsystem involvement in the environment's assessment. Because people are part of the social and cultural subsystems, the assessment function is more apparent in those components of the occupational environment. However, parameters of the physical subsystem may contribute important features that are essential for the individual to note. These physical features can markedly influence the external expectations for an occupational role. Physical attributes convey indications of both possibilities and limitations for the person in preparing and executing an occupational response designed to be adaptive and masterful. The person engaging in an occupational role requiring the use of certain equipment, for example, is both enabled and constrained by the capabilities of that equipment. The cabinet maker operates within the potentials offered by available tools. The secretary prepares documents efficiently as enabled by electronic hardware and software with its relative speed and sophistication.

Environmental stimuli, such as the ambient temperature in the workplace, call for the individual to dress for either warm or cold conditions in order to function optimally. The highway construction worker dresses differently for work under a scorching summer sun and a cold, damp winter wind. The occupational therapist whose daily activity involves assisting with physical transfer of clients with disabilities will wear shoes that provide comfort and stability on the particular transfer surfaces with which the feet come in contact. The therapist whose function involves the use of leather stains, ceramic glazes, or copper tooling chemicals will be aware of artistic possibilities and potentially harmful effects of dealing with these substances. The therapist who is responsible for clients on a community outing will want to know features of terrain, accessibility, and street patterns to lead those clients on a therapeutically successful event. Awareness of the physical features of the occupational environment is critical for the person preparing an occupational response.

The physical subsystem gives feedback to the individual regarding the satisfactory or unsatisfactory nature of the response. Persons who fail to note boundaries or hazards present in the physical or nonhuman aspects of the external expectations may place themselves at risk for personal harm at worst, and lack of success in responding to the challenge at best. The feedback is frequently instantaneous, such as a tennis serve placed very precisely within the opponent's court so as to prevent a return or a cut on the finger from an unexpectedly sharp paring knife.

The social subsystem gives feedback regarding the extent to which expectations or limitations of the social structure in a particular occupational environment have been met, respected, or violated. When the expectations are clearly delineated, the person's task in meeting those expectations is more easily perceived. In many occupational environments, the social expectations, particularly within informal social structures, may be difficult to identify and plan for. The person who is new to a particular setting will certainly encounter feedback that indicates how accurately the social subsystem is being perceived and how successfully it is negotiated. Long-standing social subsystems may be powerful influences and difficult to penetrate for the person wishing to become a part of that subsystem. The high school student, new to the community and the school, will receive clear indications of the extent to which the "welcome mat" is being laid out by the existing social subsystem. Early social interactions in the occupational role of student bring feedback regarding success or failure respective to the expectations of the social subsystem. Likewise, the new employee desiring to be a part of a social subsystem may find that it is difficult to be included·in informal gatherings of that social subsystem. This can be particularly true of those gatherings that have become ritualized, such as a group of individuals whose social activities take place over lunch or similar break periods. For a particular occupational environment, awareness of the social subsystem and its properties has the potential to substantially impact one's experience of relative mastery.

The cultural subsystem can provide some of the most powerful feedback regarding the occupational response. The rules, regulations, customs, mores, values, codes regarding ethics and behavior, policies, procedures, etc., are filled with information for the individual desiring to perform adaptively and masterfully. They constitute the "rules of the road." These rules of the road relate to the reason for the environment's existence (i.e., its mission). This is true whether the context be work or school, leisure or self-care. If education is the mission, as in school settings, there are cultural features that describe the standards and expectations for those engaged in various roles. If manufacture of a product is the mission, the culture will differ from one workplace to another. For example, a worker engaged in the manufacture of computer chips will encounter a very different culture from the one engaged in the manufacture of steel. In leisure environments, cultures likewise differ. Participation in a softball game involves cultural expectations quite different from those seen in a game of chess. The various components of an occupational environment's culture will, in part, be historical or traditional. Some will develop as a result of pressures from outside the environment, which impact the ways in which the culture operates (e.g., laws, standards of regulating bodies, or funding sources). Others emerge from the need for a group of individuals to go about tasks in a systematic or organized manner in order to achieve mission-related goals. Regardless of the make-up of a particular environmental culture, mindful attention to cultural expectations is essential if the individual is to experience a positive relative mastery. As with the social subsystem, there are "keepers" of the culture who will provide feedback to the individual regarding the degree to which the cultural expectations are being met.

All three subsystems of the occupational environment—physical, social, and cultural—evaluate (give feedback regarding) the individual's occupational response. That evaluation feeds back into the occupational environment and becomes incorporated there.

INCORPORATION INTO THE OCCUPATIONAL ENVIRONMENT

Just as evaluation of the occupational event by the individual can impact the individual and result in change (adaptation), evaluation of the same occupational event by the occupational environment has the potential for the individual's actions to effect change in the environment itself. It is at the incorporation point, the last step in the process within the occupational environment element of occupational adaptation, that the individual's impact on the occupational environment can be seen. This impact is in the form of influence on the occupational role expectations that are external to the individual. As a result of the individual acting on and within the occupational environment, the role expectations may be subject to change. The expectations may be relaxed in some manner; or, conversely, they may be reinforced or intensified. Requirements may be added or subtracted. It is also a possibility that there is no change and the individual will deal with familiar expectations when encountering or selecting subsequent occupational challenges within that particular context.

For the therapist to intervene effectively in the client's occupational life, knowledge of the occupational environment in which the client functions is critical. Thinking about this context as physical, social, and cultural in nature gives the therapist a framework for learning about the client's occupational environment and the form, intensity, and character of the expectations that impact a particular client.

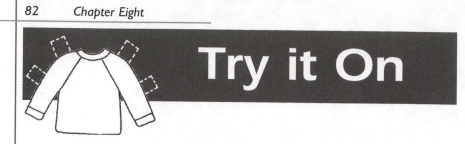

Try it On

In this final Try it On segment we are going to ask you to identify specific components of the occupational environment related to the same occupational challenge you've been working on, and then reflect on how you and the environment have interacted together.

Before we move on, let's have a brief review of the occupational environment and its role in the occupational adaptation process.

Occupational environment:
- Comprised of physical, social, and cultural influences.
- Has inherent demands for mastery.
- Has external role expectations for the person's performance.
- Involves evaluation of the person's occupational response.
- Has potential to make changes in external role expectations.

The following questions will refer you back to your occupational challenge:

Evaluation by the Occupational Environment	Comments
How did the occupational environment evaluate your response?	

Incorporation into the Occupational Environment	Comments
As a result of the environment's evaluation, what alterations would you make, if any, when engaged with the same challenge?	

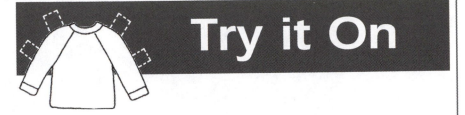

Congratulations on a job well done! While we have prompted you to "freeze-frame" components of the occupational adaptation process throughout this guide, please keep in mind that this process is dynamic and fluid.

CHAPTER NINE

What Does the Therapist Do?

Go to the people
Work with them
Learn from them
Respect them
Start with what they know
Build with what they have.
And when the work is done
The task accomplished
The people will say,
"We have done this ourselves."

Lao Tsu, China, 700 BC

In any therapeutic relationship, the occupational therapist has several important therapeutic tools to use regardless of the particular frame of reference that guides the therapist's thinking. The therapist who practices from an occupational adaptation perspective uses all of those familiar tools, as well as some others. Let's talk first about three familiar ones that every therapist has learned, then we will talk more specifically about how the therapist functions from an occupational adaptation point of view.

One obviously important tool for any intervention is *knowledge base*— knowledge of person system structures and how they interrelate and function in the service of occupation. The therapist must understand how dysfunction in these interrelated structures affects dysfunction in occupational performance. This is where a thorough understanding of activity analysis comes into play. In other words, what are the sensorimotor, cognitive, and psychosocial requirements of occupational performance in general? This knowledge tool is the basis from which you apply general knowledge to particular clients in specific instances.

Therapeutic *bag of tricks* is a second important tool. This includes various evaluations, intervention techniques, knowledge of assistive aids, ability to identify the need for environmental modifications, etc. The therapist must know whether or when it is appropriate to use them.

Third, every therapist learned during OT education that *therapeutic use of self* is an extremely important tool. In other words, as a therapist you need the ability to position yourself physically, cognitively, and psychosocially to facilitate your client's progress. You must be able to facilitate your client's progress through your carefully developed intervention plan. You must also be positioned to respond to unplanned and unexpected events in such a way as to be therapeutic. You must be attuned to information the client provides that was not a part of your assessment but surfaced naturally during the course of therapeutic interactions.

For the therapist who wishes to practice from an occupational adaptation perspective, the three tools just described are required. However, there are some additional tools that are necessary.

First and foremost you will need *an understanding of the concepts and their relationships* (i.e., how the occupational adaptation process works). Occupational adaptation is not a technique or a set of techniques. It is a way of thinking about your client and about how you approach your task as a therapist. Focus of intervention is always on the client and a client-selected occupational role.

Second, occupational adaptation tells you *what questions to ask*, not what to "do." The questions do not change from client to client. However, the answers will be very different from client to client. Once the client provides you with answers, then you begin to plan your intervention using the client-selected occupational role. Remember that dysfunction is always relative to the occupational role. If you have identified a deficit in the person systems (sensorimotor, cognitive, or psychosocial) that does not relate to the occupational role, do not mess with it! Likewise, if a particular deficit (e.g., range of motion limitation) does not interfere with the occupational performance that the client has selected, do not mess with it! Similarly, the same deficit may impact occupational performance differently from one client to the other. One size does not fit all in this case. A pianist and a forklift operator with the "same" deficit in finger mobility have different therapeutic needs.

Third, *the client/therapist relationship in occupational adaptation must be a collaborative one.* Your goal is that the client will serve as his or her own change agent. Your task is not to take away that function from the client. This is very important, because in occupational adaptation you are always trying to facilitate the client's internal adaptation capabilities. If you do not let the client exercise the choices of a self-changing agent, how can you expect the client's internal adaptation capabilities to be enhanced or strengthened? The answer is a "no-brainer"—you can't!

Nevertheless, you still have a very important role to play. Your task is to serve as the agent of the environment in which the client's occupational role is carried out. In other words, you have to set the stage for the client to carry out his or her role-related tasks just as the environment does when the client is in his or her usual surroundings or context.

What exactly does it mean to be the "agent of the occupational environment?" First of all, you have to learn what the demands of that environment are relative to the occupational role. (Remember the *demand for mastery* and the *occupational role expectations?*) Very often, these demands and expectations are something with which you may not be familiar. There may be economic influences, social influences, cultural influences, family influences, etc., that determine how the client is expected to perform. You must be willing to place yourself in the role of "learner" and allow the client to become the "teacher." Otherwise, how can you possibly plan relevant intervention? In addition, allowing the client to teach you is a wonderful empowerment tool in permitting the client to serve as a self-changing agent!

The blend of knowledge base, bag of tricks, therapeutic use of self, understanding of occupational adaptation concepts, knowing what questions to ask, and engaging in a collaborative relationship all come together to promote *the client's adaptive capacity.* The case of the Pianist gives an example of how a therapist utilized all of her therapeutic skills to engage the client in an intervention approach that was consistent with occupational adaptation principles.

THE PIANIST

Mrs. Evans was a patient in an acute psychiatric unit with a diagnosis of schizophrenia. She had been hospitalized on many occasions. A review of her chart indicated that she had very limited social interaction and refused most groups. The occupational therapist (an OT student) went to the patient's room to interview her. She found Mrs. Evans in a dark room with the lights off, curtains closed, and the bed covers pulled over her head. Mrs. Evans was uneasy about the therapist but agreed to answer a few questions. After about 4 minutes, Mrs. Evans "dismissed" the therapist but was rather polite.

During the short interview, the therapist noted that Mrs. Evans had long painted fingernails with chipped polish, dyed jet-black hair, and considerable make-up. The therapist had limited information from the interview itself, but her observations led her to believe that appearance was important to Mrs. Evans. The therapist located shades of fingernail polish from various staff members and returned to Mrs. Evans' room, inquiring if she would like to re-do her nails. Mrs. Evans was interested but did not want to go to the day room to do it. However, she did so.

Mrs. Evans opened up to the therapist as she painted her nails, with the assistance of the therapist. During this time, Mrs. Evans revealed that she had studied art and music in college and taught piano for many years. She had four children. She had grown up on a farm where she had developed a love of horseback riding. However, it had been a number of years since she had engaged in the activities she enjoyed.

Mrs. Evans lived in an assisted living environment where there was no longer a piano available. Together, Mrs. Evans and the therapist worked on identifying places in the community where she could have access to a piano. Mrs. Evans attended AA meetings weekly at a church where there was a piano. The therapist helped Mrs. Evans identify the appropriate person from whom to gain permission to use the piano and how he might be contacted. Mrs. Evans also identified other places in the community where she could try to locate a piano.

The therapist gained permission to take Mrs. Evans off the unit to a location in the hospital where there was a piano. When she sat down to play, staff members from offices along the hallway came out to see who was playing so beautifully. Later, the therapist brought music books and sheet music for Mrs. Evans to select to take home. She was excited about being able to play again.

Mrs. Evans also started coming to task group and began participating in other groups that were addressing other goals.

Case contributed by Catherine Evich Johnson, OTS

The case of the Pianist demonstrates how a therapist used all of the necessary tools from an occupational adaptation perspective.

1. She saw indications that the client still desired mastery (inferred from her appearance).
2. She identified an occupational role that was meaningful (pianist).
3. She served as the agent of the occupational environment (set the stage for the client to engage in her occupation).
4. Most importantly, she collaborated with the client, allowing the client to become her own agent of change (identifying strategies the client could use to create piano-playing opportunities).

The therapist facilitated adaptiveness in the client that would enhance her ability to engage in her preferred occupation.

Another case, that of the Woodworker (see next page) demonstrates how the therapist practicing from an occupational adaptation perspective approaches intervention.

The Woodworker is an excellent example of how an occupational therapist practicing from occupational adaptation "tunes in" to the information regarding personally meaningful occupation provided by her client and then capitalizes on that information to achieve a successful therapeutic outcome. It also demonstrates how in the "physical dysfunction" setting, it was her attention to the heavy psychosocial content of his communication that led to his engagement in intervention. She placed him in a situation where he was the "expert" by allowing him to teach her about the Dremel and permitting him to critique her technique.

This skillful therapist used all of the principles discussed in this chapter: knowledge base, techniques, therapeutic use of self, understanding of occupational adaptation, asking therapeutically appropriate questions, and engaging Mr. Robinson in a collaborative relationship with her. When the therapist takes this approach, the results can meet the needs of all parties concerned in the rehabilitation effort. The goals of the referring physician were met; the facility's need to provide effective services was met; and most importantly, Mr. Robinson's need to be rehabilitated in a therapeutic climate where his views, values, and talent were respected was met. The outcome was satisfying to both client and therapist.

THE WOODWORKER

Mr. Robinson was a 62-year-old male hospitalized for rehabilitation secondary to deconditioning. The deconditioning was the result of a complex medical history that included hypertension, a myocardial infarction, and a quadruple arterial bypass procedure.

Prior to initial assessment by occupational therapy, other rehabilitation staff reported Mr. Robinson as noncompliant, with refusal to get out of bed or perform exercises. At initial interview, Mr. Robinson reported that he was retired from the Air Force. He also reported that he had actively participated in a health club, walking and exercising daily with his spouse. Additionally, he reported a "hobby" of woodworking. His home included a wood shop in which he built grandfather clocks, furniture, and other intricate pieces. His affect clearly brightened when discussing his woodworking. Mr. Robinson indicated that he wanted to return to his previous activity level of independence in ADLs and exercise at the health club, as well as woodworking. He had shortness of breath and fatigue throughout the interview and needed to return from sitting upright to supine after 15 minutes. At the conclusion of the interview, it was mutually agreed upon that Mr. Robinson would assess a new Dremel (Racine, WI) that was recently acquired by the therapist and explain its various parts and functions.

The following day, Mr. Robinson sat on the side of the bed for 20 minutes in the morning and 30 minutes in the afternoon while enthusiastically reaching for various accessories of the Dremel and explaining their purposes. (Mr. Robinson continued to refuse physical therapy's requests to get out of bed and exercise or to go to the gym for group exercise.)

On the second day, the OT brought wood and asked Mr. Robinson if he would like to make something. He replied, "No, but I would love to show you how to use the Dremel." The therapist then suggested that he get out of bed and into a wheelchair so they could go the gym for the instruction. Mr. Robinson then donned his robe with minimum assistance, transferred to the chair with contact guard, and went to the gym.

Mr. Robinson carefully scanned the environment of the gym, observing other patients and activities. In a quiet room off of the gym, Mr. Robinson sat in the wheelchair while drawing designs on wood and demonstrating use of the Dremel. When fatigued, he would have

continued on next page

The Woodworker, continued

the therapist use the Dremel and then inspect her work. Mr. Robinson tolerated being out of bed in the wheelchair for 30 minutes in the morning and 30 minutes in the afternoon.

During this session, the therapist and Mr. Robinson discussed his heart attack that had led to the bypass procedure, and the fears and anxieties he had about resuming activity. In addition, before, during, and after each session, oxygen saturation levels were taken and recorded by Mr. Robinson following initial instruction on oximeter use. The therapist pointed out increased tolerance of activity as evidenced by gains in sitting tolerance, standing tolerance, and time out of bed.

The following morning, Mr. Robinson was dressed and ready to go to the gym for another Dremel lesson. (He still refused to participate in individual or group exercise.) This time the therapist asked Mr. Robinson to stand at the counter to do the demonstration and critique the therapist's use of the tool. Mr. Robinson tolerated standing for the lesson for 15 minutes, a 10-minute rest in his chair, and then another 15 minutes standing. During the lesson Mr. Robinson asked, "Did you hear it?" The therapist replied, "Hear what?" Mr. Robinson said, "Why, the sound of the wood talking to you." He pointed out that when the tool cut through various grains of wood, the sounds varied with the hardness of the wood. Mr. Robinson clearly loved his work with wood, was highly knowledgeable about woodworking, and easily engaged in this familiar and comfortable activity.

In the afternoon, Mr. Robinson stated that he would like to try some exercising in the gym. He did some lower and upper extremity exercises (without weights or resistance, and no upper extremity movements over 90 degrees). The following morning Mr. Robinson participated in the full rehabilitation program and continued to be active and "in compliance" through discharge and outpatient rehabilitation.

Case reported by Joanna Lipoma, MOT, OTR

CHAPTER TEN

How Do You Describe Occupational Adaptation to Others

Holistic

Every client has
desire for mastery

Client is the
agent of change

Client is involved
in evaluation

Now that you have worked through the occupational adaptation process for yourself in the Try it On exercises, you are ready to focus on how to introduce and explain the process to others. We have had successful outcomes and positive feedback with the following approaches in both academic and clinical settings. Our experience as clinicians and educators has taught us the importance of being able to articulate what we're doing that makes us "different" from others. As you have experienced for yourself in this book, practicing from this framework is distinctively different than other frequently used perspectives in the clinical arena. Let's discuss the different case scenarios that you might experience and the strategy of "telling it like it is" to various audiences.

THE PHYSICIAN

We all know that the physician's time is limited. We need to address issues quickly and concisely, "get in and get out" as we tell our occupational therapy interns. Whether you are selling occupational therapy for an initial consult or rationalizing your approach to treatment, the major assumptions of occupational adaptation are the ticket in this situation. They have been threaded throughout the guide and re-emphasized here.

Holistic

While there are many disciplines using this term, it is important that you take a few moments to explain how your approach addresses the whole person system: sensorimotor, cognitive, and psychosocial. It has been our experience that in a "physical dysfunction" setting, physicians have been surprised that occupational therapy addresses more than the sensorimotor. This is why in treatment team meetings, the occupational therapist practicing from an occupational adaptation perspective reports on patients' cognition and psychosocial responses while engaged in ADLs or other occupational tasks. Likewise, in "psychiatric" settings, the physicians have been enlightened that occupational therapy is incorporating sensorimotor and cognitive functions when seeing patients. This explains why the occupational therapist practicing from an occupational adaptation theoretical perspective is not limiting services to paper and pencil counseling sessions but including other client-meaningful activities to remediate sensorimotor and cognitive deficits.

The Client is the Agent of Change

Remember that the typical physician population comes from the traditional medical model. They are used to doing procedures *to* their clients, and/or prescribing drugs that the patient takes to facilitate an internal chemical change. Historically, a patient under a physician's care does not question the recommended treatment and/or medicine being prescribed. Therefore, it is essential that you describe how your approach focuses on empowering the *client* to be the agent of change, while *you* the occupational therapist are active in "setting the stage" by designing the environment for client adaptation to occur. It is oftentimes at this point that the physician understands patient reports of doing "strange" activities in occupational therapy sessions, such as flower arranging, fishing with hip wader boots, etc., all of which are performed with "real" materials. We find that physicians often ask,"How did you know how to do that? Do you fish in the swamps?" This is the perfect opening to boast about our patients' involvement in designing their own occupational therapy treatment challenges. Not to mention, this involvement requires the patient to engage a great deal of cognitive effort to teach the occupational therapist about fishing in the swamps!

Belief That Every Client Has a Desire for Mastery

Briefly describe how you believe that every client (use *their* client as an example) has a desire to master something. We have found that stating our "trick of the trade" is the client's primary occupational role and we go from there. We often reiterate at this point that those clients, being agents and directors of their own occupational therapy challenges, get "fired up" to master the activities that the occupational therapist provides. Isn't it true that when our patients are engaged in activities they *want* to master, they give their *best* effort?

The Client is Involved With the Environment in the Evaluation Process

Physicians need to know that the "secret of your success" is that the patient and occupational therapist collaboratively and dynamically evaluate the patient's response to the challenges being addressed in occupational therapy. The treatment process from initial assessment through discharge is formulated and altered by the clients' evaluation of whether or not they feel they are efficient, effective, and satisfied with their progress and performance.

THE CLINICAL COMMUNITY

This category of individuals was hard to name, because we find ourselves describing our approach to clinicians of other disciplines on the team, as well as other occupational therapists. Therefore, we will approach this category encompassing all clinicians on the team. In our experience, the inquiries we receive about our approach to occupational therapy treatment are based on a treatment session they observe, or ones in which they are directly involved (such as co-treatment sessions or team teaching), and/or feedback they hear from others. Using the "client in question" is the way to go. Use the specific case/class/client as the base for your description. We will usually describe our approach using the general occupational adaptation assumptions, then go directly to the particular client and the client's primary occupational role. Description of the initiated treatment program then follows naturally. This is an excellent opportunity to put meaning for others into what is being used to reach occupational therapy goals. We also explain what activities the occupational therapist is using as readiness and what challenges the client is engaged in that are occupational activities for *that* individual. This usually ends up with a discussion of why our clients do not all do the same thing, even if they have a similar diagnosis and/or primary physician.

Often in treatment team meetings, we have had the experience of being consulted to offer suggestions for how to deal with a "difficult" client, or one that is "unmotivated" for therapy. Our usual response is, "Did you ask the client what he or she wants to do?" This is an automatic response from us because of the inherent assumption in occupational adaptation that the person has a desire to master *something*. Finding this *something* is what makes treatment so dynamic and individualistic. Telling it like it is involves educating others about the process and approach to treatment but also educating them on how to use the occupational adaptation approach in involving the client. It is not a novel concept to include the client in the evaluative process, but is often overlooked and underemphasized. So, next time a fellow team member is brainstorming about what to do next with an "unmotivated" or "uncooperative" client, try asking what it is the client desires to do and whether that is being threaded into the therapeutic process. Part of our reward as occupational therapists practicing the occupational adaptation theory has been not only being a part of the relative mastery that our patients experience, but also witnessing the relative mastery other team members experience when they can focus on their patients' primary occupational role, use it in treatment, and reap the rewards for their efforts!

THE OCCUPATIONAL THERAPIST

This final section addresses the "inquiring mind" of the occupational therapist population. Often, occupational therapists know the basics of the occupational adaptation framework and have heard general information about it. They often have case scenarios of their own that map on to some of the cases presented or documented in publications. Their comments generally range from, "This sounds like what I do," to "Isn't this what occupational therapy is all about?" It is at this point that these questions be answered in-depth with the components of the occupational adaptation framework. Yes, it does require an element of time. Can you imagine if we attempted to engage you in the adaptive response subprocesses in one chapter in this book? Keep in mind that sufficiently answering questions from the inquisitive occupational therapist takes time. How much time does it take? We will attempt to separate and give suggestions for the common avenues that we have used.

The Inservice

Most occupational therapy departments have times set aside for staff inservices. This may be during a weekly staff meeting or a designated inservice time. Typically, allotted time is about 1 hour, maybe less. This is not a tremendous amount of time to delve into the adaptive response subprocesses. Keep it simple—explain the major assumptions of occupational adaptation with emphasis on its uniqueness. Use a handout and/or transparency of the schematic to identify the person, occupational environment, and interaction of these as challenges occur. We have found that providing a case example then plugging that person into the schematic for explanation is beneficial. Do not be surprised if you get an invitation from the group to come back to explain further.

The Short Course or Workshop

The short course or workshop gives more time to really get into the occupational adaptation process. Initial time should be set aside to lay the foundation for the occupational adaptation framework. This includes history, assumptions, and unique characteristics of the theory. Next, describe the person and the occupational environment with specifics of the assumptions and components. We always have participants complete a short exercise illustrating these foundational concepts on themselves. The following time should be spent according to the people present in your short course or workshop. We will explain two methods, each having their own strengths.

If you get the feeling that your group participants are game for a challenge and can wait awhile for a description of the role of the occupational therapist, then address the person first. This next chunk of time needs to be devoted to the three adaptive response subprocesses (generation, evaluation, and integration). This is our favorite part, as we believe the unique flavor of this theory really comes alive when you begin to explore these. Have your participants engage in applying these concepts through short group activities, discussions, and/or paper description. We have found that participants seem to integrate more easily when relating to a personal example before applying the theory to a patient. Finish with the occupational environment and its role in the occupational adaptation process. The second way to delve into the occupational adaptation process after explaining the general assumptions and description of the person and occupational environment is to begin with the occupational environment. Why? We advocate beginning with the occupational environment when the group participants are pressing for "how" and "what role does the occupational therapist play?" It is similar to the first method; however, you are beginning with the occupational environment and then following with the person and adaptive processes. Again, the method you use will depend on the group attending. Either way, it is always wise to finish your short course or workshop with time to explore a case and answer questions to sum up the experience.

The Institute/All-Day Workshop

As the title of this section suggests, you have more time to illustrate the flow of the occupational adaptation process. We would suggest group activities to facilitate understanding of the main occupational adaptation framework. Having an all-day workshop also gives the participants time to use the framework personally and professionally. Participation from the audience for examples of the occupational adaptation process "at work" in patient care is typically very contagious. Do not forget to allot time to describe/update the research being developed and documented with occupational adaptation. This book will help with references, etc. Do not be afraid to write up some of your patient cases and use them as scenarios for discussion. It can be a great learning experience for you and the group participants. Consult the cases in this book for examples of how you might develop your application of occupational adaptation into case studies for discussion.

BELMONT UNIVERSITY LIBRARY

BELMONT UNIVERSITY LIBRARY

Index

adaptation energy
    definition, 33-34
    levels, 35-37, 45
adaptation gestalt. *See also* adaptive response evaluation subprocess
    case study, 54-56
    exercise, 57-58
    holistic approach, 52-54, 94
    overview, 51-52
adaptive response behaviors, 34, 39-44, 45
adaptive response evaluation subprocess
    case study, 64-65
    exercise, 66
    overview, 61
    relative mastery, 62-64, 65
    self-generated responses, 32
adaptive response generation subprocess. *See also* adaptation gestalt; adaptive response integration subprocess; occupational challenge; occupational environments
    case studies, 38, 40-41, 43-44
    definition, 32
    exercises, 47-49
    overview, 31
    therapeutic perspective, 32-37, 39, 41-46
adaptive response integration subprocess
    case study, 72-73
    definition, 32
    evaluating, 70-71
    exercise, 74
    overview, 69
adaptive response mechanism, 33
adaptive response modes, 34, 37-39, 45
adrenal glands, 33
afghan maker case study, 17
"agent of the occupational environment", 87, 94-95
aversive events, 70

bag of tricks, 86

case studies
    afghan maker, 17
    chess player, 43-44
    elder homemaker, 72-73
    first-time mother, 3-4

florist, 64-65
husband caregiver, 54-56
occupational adaptation process, 3-4
pianist, 88-89
preacher, 38
researcher, 40-41
water skier, 27
woodworker, 90-91
chess player case study, 43-44
client/therapist relationship, 87
clinical community, 95-96
cognitive system, 24, 25, 53
competence, 14
cultural subsystem, 22, 24, 78-80

demand for mastery, 15
desire for mastery, 14-15, 17, 19, 95
dysadaptive response, 70

elder homemaker case study, 72-73
environmental subsystem, 24
existing adaptive response mode, 37, 39, 45
experiential/phenomenological subsystem, 24
external role expectations, 22-24

first-time mother case study, 3-4
florist case study, 64-65
"freeze-frame" approach, 4

genetic subsystem, 24, 25

hand dysfunction, 44-45
holistic approach, 52-54, 94
homemaker case study, 72-73
homeostasis, 70
husband caregiver case study, 54-56

inservices, 97
internal role expectations, 24-25
intervention, 6, 71

knowledge base, 86

leisure/play, 22
life roles, 2, 3

mastery, 13, 14-17. *See also* relative mastery
mature adaptive response behaviors, 41, 42-43, 45
modified adaptive response mode, 37, 39, 45

new adaptive response mode, 37, 39, 45
"normative" process, 2

occupational adaptation process. *See also* adaptation energy; adaptive
      response integration subprocess; occupational challenge
   case studies
      first-time mother, 3-4
      pianist, 88-89
   clinical community, 95-96
   components, 4, 8
   "cross-section" example, 4-5
   definition, 2-3
   evaluating, 71
   guide to practice, 7
   internal, 78
   intervention, 6, 8, 71
   occupational therapist's role, 96-98
   physician's role, 94-95
   therapeutic tools, 86-87
   training, 97-98
occupational adaptation theory
   definition, 1-3
occupational challenge. *See also* adaptive response generation subprocess
   case study, 27
   exercise, 28
   role expectations
      external, 22-24
      interacting, 26
      internal, 24-25
      overview, 21-22
occupational dysadaptation, 70
occupational environments
   exercise, 82-83
   external role expectations, 22-24
   overview, 77-78
   subsystems, 78-80
   therapeutic perspective, 81

person systems, 25
physical subsystem, 22, 78-80
physician, role in occupational adaptation process, 94-95
pianist case study, 88-89
play. See leisure/play
preacher case study, 38
press for mastery, 15-16
primary adaptation energy, 35-37, 45
primitive adaptive response behaviors, 41, 42, 45
psychosocial system, 24, 25, 53

relative mastery, 6, 62-64, 62-64, 65, 70. *See also* adaptive response
    integration subprocess
researcher case study, 40-41
role expectations. *See* occupational challenge

secondary adaptation energy, 35-37, 45
self-care occupational environments, 22
self-generated responses, 32
sensorimotor system, 24, 53
skill mastery, 62
social subsystem, 22, 78-80
spatiotemporal adaptation, 41
staff inservices, 97

therapeutic tools, 86-87
therapeutic use of self, 86
transitional adaptive response behaviors, 41, 42, 45

water skier case study, 27
woodworker case study, 90-91
work, 22
workshops, 97-98

BELMONT UNIVERSITY LIBRARY

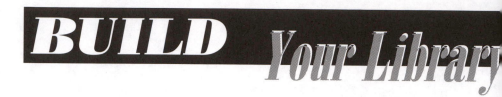

This book and many others on numerous different topics are available from SLACK Incorporated. For further information or a copy of our latest catalog, contact us at:

**Professional Book Division
SLACK Incorporated
6900 Grove Road
Thorofare, NJ 08086 USA
Telephone: 1-856-848-1000
1-800-257-8290
Fax: 1-856-853-5991
E-mail: orders@slackinc.com
www.slackbooks.com**

We accept most major credit cards and checks or money orders in US dollars drawn on a US bank. Most orders are shipped within 72 hours.

Contact us for information on recent releases, forthcoming titles, and bestsellers. If you have a comment about this title or see a need for a new book, direct your correspondence to the Editorial Director at the above address.

Thank you for your interest and we hope you found this work beneficial.

BELMONT UNIVERSITY LIBRARY

Occupational Adaptation in Practice

Concepts and Cases

Who says theory can't be fun, practical, and understandable? *Occupational Adaptation in Practice: Concepts and Cases* is a user-friendly text that clearly describes the theory of occupational adaptation.

This new text describes one approach to occupation-based, client-centered practice. The purpose of this guide is to make occupational adaptation easily understood and applied. This exceptional guide leads the reader through the flow and understanding of this theory. Practical examples help demonstrate how theory can be implemented in practice. It breaks the components of the theory into smaller, more manageable units. Included in the text are cases in which practitioners have used occupational adaptation in various practice settings.

Features

- Conversational style promotes reader understanding of the ideas in occupational adaptation

- "Try It On" feature gives the reader an opportunity to apply the concepts to a personal everyday life situation

- The guide provides the practitioner with suggestions on how to apply occupational adaptation to practice

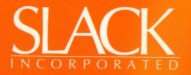

SLACK
INCORPORATED

ISBN 1-55642-553-8

90000

9 781556 425530